NHA Phlebotomy
Study Guide 2023-2024

Ace the Certified Phlebotomy Technician Exam on Your First Try with No Effort | Test Questions, Answer Keys & Tips to Score a 98% Pass Rate

Elenore Stryker

Educational Prep Academy

TABLE OF CONTENTS

Introduction

We are pleased to welcome you to the most comprehensive review resource for the Certified Phlebotomy Technician (CPT) Examination offered by the National Healthcareer Association (NHA). The National Healthcareer Association Phlebotomy Exam is approaching, and our thorough study guide is here to help you get ready for it. In it, you'll find a comprehensive introduction to the test, a wealth of information on the most important facets of phlebotomy, and helpful advice on how to effectively study for and complete the examination. This study guide is designed to be an all-encompassing resource that will provide you with everything you need to know to flourish in your phlebotomy job and pass the exam required for certification.

In the first chapter, you will learn about the National Healthcareer Association Phlebotomy Exam, its format, and what you can anticipate on the day of the test. In addition to that, it offers techniques for effective exam preparation as well as methods for overcoming test anxiety.

The function of the phlebotomist as well as the duties associated with it are discussed in Chapter 2. You will receive an in-depth awareness of the legal and ethical aspects in phlebotomy, including major regulatory criteria, as well as the necessary characteristics of a successful phlebotomist. In addition, you will study the essential characteristics of a successful phlebotomist.

In the third chapter, we examine phlebotomy-related workplace safety rules, compliance requirements, and quality assurance measures. It offers an in-depth comprehension of the significance of safety and compliance in phlebotomy practice, which is essential for the profession.

You will receive an introduction to fundamentals of human anatomy in chapter 4. This chapter offers a comprehensive explanation of the many body systems, the structure of blood, and the coagulation process, all of which are essential for the practice of phlebotomy.

In Chapter 5, we go through all of the different components of preparing a patient for phlebotomy operations, from identifying the patient and obtaining consent to discussing venipuncture equipment and choosing a location.

The equipment and procedures utilized in routine blood collection are discussed in Chapter 6. This includes the selection of devices, the order in which draws are performed, and needle safety devices.

This chapter provides information regarding pediatric volumes, peripheral blood smear collections, and blood culture collections, among other types of specialized collections in the field of phlebotomy.

Dermal puncture is the topic of discussion in Chapter 8, which also includes a comprehensive discussion of the underlying principles, supplies, and techniques.

The screening of newborns is an essential part of pediatric phlebotomy, and we will go deeper into this topic in the following chapter.

In chapter 10, a thorough review of the processing step of phlebotomy is presented. This stage includes centrifuging, aliquoting, handling, storing, transporting, and disposing of specimens.

This chapter dives into the various responsibilities of a phlebotomist besides the collection of blood, such as educating patients on the collection of specimens and managing specimens that are not blood.

The fundamental skills necessary to work as a phlebotomy technician are reviewed in Chapter 12, including the nomenclature, blood components, and pre-analytical errors that may occur.

In chapter 13, we discuss the fundamental aspects of laboratory information systems, including quality control and assurance, as well as the significance of interpersonal communication.

This chapter will test your knowledge and readiness for the NHA Phlebotomy Exam by providing you with practice questions to work through.

In Chapter 15, you will find in-depth explanations for the solutions to the practice questions that were presented in the prior chapter.

The bonus chapter will provide you with hidden keys that will make your studying more productive and your preparation for the exam more effective.

So, without any further ado, let's get started!

Chapter 1

An overview of the NHA Phlebotomy Exam

This chapter is dedicated to presenting you with an in-depth review of the Certified Phlebotomy Technician (CPT) Exam that is administered by the National Healthcareer Association (NHA). The major objective is to acquaint you with the format and material of the test, as well as what to expect on the day of the exam, as well as techniques for passing the exam, advice for effective test-taking, ways for overcoming test anxiety, and an efficient preparation strategy. By the time you reach the conclusion of this chapter, you should have a good idea of what to anticipate and how to organize yourself to achieve success.

Chapter Overview

What the Exam Consists Of

The National Healthcareer Association Certified Phlebotomy Technician Exam is an all-encompassing test that evaluates your phlebotomy knowledge and abilities. It normally contains of questions with multiple choice answers that cover a broad range of topics, including the function of the phlebotomist, the preparation of the patient, collection techniques, safety and compliance, processing and handling of specimens, and other important aspects of phlebotomy.

What to Expect on Exam Day

On the day of the exam, you need to make sure that you go to the testing site in enough of time before your allotted starting time. You will be required to produce a legitimate form of identification in addition to your exam confirmation. After you have been checked in, you will be given instructions on the policies and procedures that govern the exam, including how to utilize any permitted materials and how to manage any personal items that may arise during the course of the test. The test will most likely be administered on a computer, and you will be allotted a certain amount of time to finish it.

How To Pass The Exam

In order to succeed on the NHA CPT Exam, candidates need to possess both theoretical understanding and practical experience. It is essential to have a complete comprehension of all of the subject matter that is included in the test outline, and it is equally essential to have mastered the practical abilities through the completion of relevant on-the-job training. Regular study, knowing the test format, preparing with mock examinations, and revisiting any weak areas can significantly raise the likelihood that you will pass the exam.

Test Tips

Taking a test is always a nerve-wracking experience, but if you prepare properly, it can become less overwhelming and more bearable. Be sure to read each question thoroughly, eliminate any answers that are patently incorrect, carefully manage the time allotted to you, and maintain your composure for the entirety of the test.

How To Overcome Test Anxiety

Anxiety about how well one will perform on a test can be a substantial barrier to doing well. A number of different methods, including positive affirmations, progressive muscle relaxation, deep breathing, and visualization, can be of assistance in the management of test anxiety. In the days preceding up to the test, it is of the utmost importance to maintain a healthy lifestyle by engaging in regular physical activity, consuming a food that is nutritionally sound, and getting a enough amount of sleep.

Study Strategy

Creating an efficient plan of study is one of the most important steps in getting ready for the test. This includes creating a schedule for studying, concentrating on one subject at a time, taking breaks at regular intervals, and frequently reviewing previously learned material. In addition, practice exams can be an invaluable instrument for evaluating your level of comprehension and readiness for the examination.

Your path toward becoming a Certified Phlebotomy Technician begins with this chapter, which lays the groundwork for the rest of your studies. You will be well on your way to having a fruitful career in phlebotomy if you have an idea of what the examination comprises and how to prepare for it.

What the exam consists of

The Certified Phlebotomy Technician (CPT) Exam that is offered by the National Healthcareer Association (NHA) is an all-encompassing test that is meant to examine the candidate's knowledge, skills, and abilities necessary to successfully carry out the responsibilities of a Phlebotomy Technician. Your theoretical knowledge as well as your practical skills will be put to the test throughout the exam, which is broken up into numerous sections that reflect the actual procedure of phlebotomy in the real world.

Structure of the Exam

Typically, there are about 120 scored questions on the CPT exam, in addition to 20 pretest questions that are not scored. The total number of questions on the exam is typically close to one hundred forty, and you are typically allotted two hours to do it.

The questions are in a multiple-choice format, which means that you will need to select the appropriate response from a list of possibilities. Your ability to comprehend and apply the knowledge and skills necessary for the position of Phlebotomy Technician will be evaluated based on your performance on these exercises.

Content Areas

There are seven primary curriculum areas that are covered on the exam, all of which mirror the responsibilities of a Phlebotomy Technician. The following is a rundown of these topics, along with an estimate of how much weight each one will carry on the exam:

Safety and Compliance (15%)

Your knowledge of safety measures, infection control methods, and regulatory compliance, including adherence to standards such as the Health Insurance Portability and Accountability Act (HIPAA), will be evaluated in this section of the test.

Patient Preparation (15%)

Your competence to prepare patients for phlebotomy operations, including identifying the patient, obtaining consent, and determining the proper site for collection, will be evaluated in this section of the exam.

Routine Blood Collection (30%)

This component of the test is the longest and most in-depth, and it covers the various methods that are commonly used to draw blood, such as venipuncture and capillary collection. Your knowledge of the tools, methods, and protocols necessary to collect blood samples in a responsible and efficient manner will be evaluated here.

Special Collections and Point-of-Care Testing (10%)

In this section, you will be tested on your knowledge of specialized collection procedures and point-of-care testing, such as blood culture collection, therapeutic phlebotomy, and glucose testing performed at the bedside.

Processing and Handling of Specimens (15%)

In this section, you will be tested on your knowledge of the appropriate methods for processing, handling, and storing specimens, as well as the labeling and transportation of these items.

Non-Blood Specimens and Alternative Collection Techniques (10%)

In this section, you will be tested on your ability to collect, handle, and process non-blood specimens such as urine and feces samples, in addition to alternate collection methods such as swab collections.

Professionalism, Quality, and Communication (5%)

Within the context of the healthcare industry, your knowledge of professional conduct, quality assurance procedures, and the ability to communicate effectively will be evaluated here.

Preparation for the Exam

It is absolutely necessary to have a complete comprehension of the subject matter areas that will be tested as well as the kinds of questions that will be on the examination. An in-depth test plan, which is provided by the NHA and serves as an important resource for your preparation, is available to you. It is essential that students engage in consistent study, go through the test strategy, and practice with questions that are similar to those that will appear on the exam.

The purpose of the test is not just to assess how well you know the material, but also how effectively you are able to apply what you have learned in a real-world setting. Therefore, it is essential to supplement your theoretical studies with actual, hands-on training in phlebotomy methods in order to ensure that you are adequately prepared for the job.

Your readiness for a job as a Phlebotomy Technician will be put to the test in a manner that is both rigorous and thorough when you take the NHA CPT Exam. You will be able to effectively customize your study strategy to match the demands of the exam and eventually achieve success if you have a solid understanding of both the format and the material that will be covered on the test.

What to Expect on Exam Day

On the day of the National Healthcareer Association Certified Phlebotomy Technician (CPT)

NHA Phlebotomy Study Guide

Exam, one could feel a mixture of excitement and nervousness. If you are well-prepared and know what to anticipate, you can help ease some of the stress that you are feeling. On the day of your exam, you can normally anticipate the following things to happen:

Before Leaving Home

Start your day off right by eating a nutritious breakfast to provide yourself the mental and physical stamina you'll need to perform well on the test. Verify that you are in possession of your entry ticket, a valid form of identification (often a driver's license or passport), and any other materials that may be necessary. Be certain that you are familiar with the path to the exam location, and set out early enough to ensure that you will arrive on time.

Arriving at the Test Center

Make sure to give yourself at least a half an hour to get to the testing center before the start of your exam. You will have sufficient time to check in, orient yourself to the surroundings, and gather your thoughts before the beginning of the exam if you follow these instructions. You will be required to present both your admission ticket and an acceptable form of identification when you arrive.

Check-In Process

During the process of checking in, the staff at the test center will verify your identity, register you for the test, and go over the policies and procedures of the test facility with you. You will be asked to store any personal goods, such as bags, electronic devices, and study materials, in a designated area, as these items are normally not permitted in the testing room. If you bring any of these items with you, you will be asked to leave them there.

The Testing Room

The examination space is typically calm, well-lit, and furnished with computers for the purpose of the test. At each workstation, there will be a partition installed to help reduce the number of interruptions. An administrator at the testing center will provide you with a seat assignment. After you have been seated, a quick lesson on how to use the computer and how to navigate through the exam will be given to you.

During the Exam

The NHA CPT Exam is normally a test that is administered on a computer and consists of questions with multiple choice answers. The test will give you a total of two hours to finish it. In order to assist you in time management, a countdown timer will be displayed on the screen of the computer. If you finish the test early, you will have the opportunity to go back and look over your answers before turning it in.

The software that administers the test might have a "mark" function that lets you indicate which questions you do not fully understand. This function might be helpful for organizing your time and ensuring that you respond to each question in the survey.

Breaks and Emergencies

During the NHA CPT Exam, there are typically no scheduled breaks that are allowed. If you feel that you need to take a break, you are free to do so without first requesting permission. However, the timer for the exam will continue to run even as you take a break.

In the event of a critical situation, immediately contact the administrator of the testing center. They will be able to direct you through the essential steps.

After the Exam

After you have finished the test, you are to leave the room in which it is being administered in a discreet manner. You will receive information from the administrator of the testing center regarding the timing and procedure for receiving your results.

The day of your exam may be stressful, but if you have adequately prepared for it and are aware of what to anticipate, you will be able to get through it with confidence. Be sure you obtain a full night's sleep, drink enough of water, and retain a cheerful attitude in the hours leading up to the test. Keep in mind that the time you spent preparing has provided you with the information and practice you need to be successful. Good luck!

How To Pass The Exam

Becoming a certified phlebotomy technician requires passing the Certified Phlebotomy Technician (CPT) exam administered by the National Healthcareer Association (NHA). The following are some suggestions for how to go in order to accomplish this.

Understand the Exam Structure and Content

Learning the format and material of the test is the first step towards doing well on it. Learn what will be covered on the test and what kinds of questions will be asked. The NHA offers a thorough study guidance in the form of a test schedule.

Create a Study Plan

The key to exam success is establishing a regular study routine. Divide the material up into more manageable bits and set aside dedicated study time for each section. Make sure you spend equal time learning both theory and practise. Keep tabs on your study schedule and make adjustments as you go along.

Master the Theoretical Knowledge

Many other areas, including as patient and worker safety, blood collection techniques, specimen processing, and professional conduct, are tested on the CPT exam. To learn more about these subjects, use textbooks, the internet, and study guides. Make sure you fully grasp the concepts underlying each method and the reasoning behind any suggested best practises.

Develop Your Practical Skills

The exam is a combination of academic knowledge and the ability to perform phlebotomy procedures in a clinical setting. Take part in practical exercises to hone your new abilities and boost your self-assurance. Practise the methods frequently so that they become automatic.

Use Practice Tests

The value of practise tests for learning for an examination cannot be overstated. You can use them to gauge your level of preparation, pinpoint areas in which you need more work, and monitor your progress towards the real thing. Prepare for the exam by taking as many practise examinations as possible.

Review and Reinforce

The best way to remember information is to revisit it frequently. Practise making it a habit to review material you've already learned. To improve your memory, try active recall methods like quizzing yourself or educating others.

Take Care of Your Health

Your health, both mental and physical, has a big impact on how well you do on tests. Make sure you're getting enough sleep, exercising regularly, and keeping a healthy diet. These routines can give you more oomph, help you focus, and calm you down.

Manage Your Time Effectively

Managing your time wisely is a must for passing the exam. You can enhance your speed and accuracy by training under timed settings. Keep track of time during the actual exam and work efficiently to guarantee that you get through every question.

Stay Calm and Focused

Worrying about how you'll perform on a test is counterproductive. Learn to deal with stress in healthy ways by implementing techniques like deep breathing, progressive muscle relaxation, and affirmations of hope. Keep your cool, pay attention in class, and have faith in your preparation on the day of the exam.

Understand the Scoring System

You can better prepare for the exam by learning the grading scheme. For instance, it is preferable to guess an answer rather than leave a question blank if there is no penalty for giving the wrong one.

Review and Learn From Mistakes

Review your practise test results and figure out where you went wrong. You can avoid making the same mistakes on the real exam if you study and reflect on your practise tests.

Prepare well, use efficient study methods, and maintain a positive outlook to succeed on the NHA CPT Exam. If you put in the time and effort and adopt the appropriate approach, you will pass the exam and take a major step forward in your phlebotomy career.

Test Tips

It's not easy to be ready for and then pass the Certified Phlebotomy Technician (CPT) Exam. However, you may maximise your performance and boost your chances of passing with the appropriate attitude and tactics. Here are some helpful hints for the exam:

Understand the Exam Structure and Content

Know the format of the test, the amount of questions, the time allotted, and the primary subject areas before you begin studying. The NHA provides a comprehensive test schedule that can be used as a helpful study tool.

Develop a Study Schedule

Make a study plan that will allow you to fully prepare for the exam's material. Set aside time to discuss each subject and stick to your schedule. Consistent, regular study periods are preferable than frantic, last-minute preparation.

Use Multiple Study Resources

Avoid relying solely on any one study tool. Learn from a variety of sources, including traditional textbooks, online tutorials, study aids, and flashcards. Using a variety of resources to learn about a topic is an excellent approach to learn the material thoroughly.

Take Practice Tests

One of the most helpful study strategies is taking practise examinations. They get you used to the exam environment, point out your weak spots, and allow you to monitor your progress. Take the time to check over your test results and figure out where you went wrong.

Master the Basics

Make sure you have a solid understanding of phlebotomy's foundational ideas. If you know the basics, you'll have a better chance of solving more complicated problems that call for application or analysis.

Understand Key Procedures

Know how to properly identify patients, choose appropriate sites, perform venipunctures, and handle specimens. You should be able to detail these processes and justify their significance.

Learn the Terminology

Phlebotomists use a unique lexicon in the course of their work. Learn the meanings of some frequent phlebotomy terminology. This can improve your comprehension of the questions and the quality of your responses to them.

Manage Your Time

Time yourself during the exam and work steadily to ensure you get through every question. Don't waste too much time trying to solve a challenging question. Put a tick next to it and move on to the following item. If you have time, you can revisit the issue at a later date.

Read the Questions Carefully

Before responding, please give each question a thorough reading. Keep an eye out for phrases and words that could play a role in the response.

Trust Your First Instinct

Your initial impressions are often the most accurate. If you can't put your finger on the right answer, go with your instinct unless there's a strong reason to do otherwise.

Stay Calm

Don't lose your cool during the test. If you find yourself becoming apprehensive or worried, tell yourself that you have done everything possible to ensure your success.

Take Care of Your Health

Your health, both mental and physical, has a direct bearing on how well you do on tests. In the days preceding up to the test, it is especially important to maintain a nutritious diet, engage in regular exercise, and get plenty of rest.

Review and Reflect

Spend some time thinking about how you could have done better on the exam. Even if you do well on the exam, it is still beneficial to analyse your performance and learn from your mistakes so that you can become a better phlebotomy technician in the future.

Keep in mind that the purpose of the CPT Exam is to assess more than just your knowledge, but also your ability to apply that knowledge in the actual world. You can feel prepared and confident on test day if you combine smart study techniques with real-world experience.

How To Overcome Test Anxiety

No matter how well you've studied or how well you know the material, everyone might experience test anxiety. It manifests itself in ways that make it difficult to do well on an exam, such as excessive concern, nervousness, or uncomfortable. If you suffer from test anxiety, try these methods:

Preparation and Organization

Being well-prepared is one of the best methods to manage exam anxiety. Make a study plan and stick to it so that you may finish studying for the test with plenty of time to spare. Being well-prepared and well-organized can help you feel more at ease.

Understand the Test Format

Learn the test's structure, such as the number of questions, time limit, and grading system. Having an idea of what will be on the test will help you relax and get in the zone.

Practice Deep Breathing and Relaxation Techniques

Relax your nervous system and lessen your anxiousness by practising deep breathing exercises. Get in the habit of breathing deeply and slowly via your nose and out your mouth. Stress and anxiety can be reduced with the use of other relaxation techniques as well, such as progressive muscle relaxation or visualisation.

Maintain a Healthy Lifestyle

Stress can be reduced and mental performance enhanced by regular exercise, a healthy diet, and sufficient sleep. Try to work exercise into your regular schedule, eat healthily, and get plenty of sleep in the days leading up to the exam.

Positive Self-Talk

Keep an upbeat disposition and talk to yourself in a positive way. Think about your skills and how hard you've worked to get ready for the test. You should try to replace negative self-talk like "I can't do this" with more positive statements like "I've prepared for this, and I can do it."

Practice Mindfulness and Meditation

Being mindful means paying attention to the here and now without passing judgement on it. If you can keep yourself from dwelling on what might happen, you may feel less anxious. The mind can be stilled and concentration sharpened by meditative practise.

Take Regular Breaks During Study

Long periods of study without rest can cause fatigue and stress. Take frequent, brief breaks from your studying. Take this opportunity to do some light stretching, go for a stroll, or do something else calming.

Practice Under Exam Conditions

Try to recreate the testing conditions in your practise sessions. In a calm, distraction-free setting, you can time yourself as you respond to sample questions or complete sample tests. This might get you used to the flow of the exam and ease your nerves.

Seek Support

Do not put off getting help if your anxiety becomes unbearable. One such source is a group or individual therapy session. Anxiety can be reduced by talking about your concerns and receiving supportive feedback.

Use Anxiety-Reducing Techniques on Exam Day

Make sure you give yourself plenty of time to get to the testing site and settle in without feeling rushed. Use positive self-talk and deep breathing exercises to help you calm down before the test begins. If you start to feel nervous while taking the exam, stop, breathe deeply, and regroup.

Celebrate Your Efforts

Remember to enjoy the process as much as the result. Recognising the time and effort you put into studying and taking an exam is crucial.

A mix of effective studying strategies, stress management methods, and a confident outlook can help students overcome test anxiety. Keep in mind that test-day jitters are completely normal and, in fact, beneficial. But if your worry is getting in the way of your work, you should try some of the methods indicated above or go to a specialist.

Study Strategy

Planning, self-discipline, and an awareness of your own learning style are the three pillars of an effective study plan. Listed below are methods to help you study more efficiently and effectively:

Set Clear Goals

Establish your study objectives and make sure they are realistic and attainable. Every objective needs to be SMART, or well-defined, reasonable, attainable, and time-bound. This method aids with concentration and boosts morale as successes are accrued along the way.

Understand Your Learning Style

Everyone has a unique way of taking in information. There are those who learn best through seeing, others through hearing, and still others through doing (kinesthetic learners). Learn how you best retain information and implement strategies to maximize that style.

Create a Study Schedule

Setting aside time each day to study helps establish consistency. Schedule your study sessions during times of the day when you know you'll be at your most awake and focused. Maintain a regular study routine.

Break It Down

Dissect complicated issues into more manageable chunks. Breaking up your studying into manageable portions has been shown to increase both understanding and retention.

Use Active Learning Strategies

Learning occurs when students actively participate in the process, rather than when they merely consume the material. Learning outcomes may include paraphrasing, instructing others, or using knowledge in practical situations.

Use a Variety of Study Materials

Don't put all your faith in literature. Make good use of study aids like study groups, flashcards, online tutorials, and practice examinations. Having a variety of resources to study from can both improve retention and keep you from getting bored.

Practice Testing

Frequent practice tests are an excellent way to solidify your knowledge and recall of the topic. As a bonus, it will get you used to the exam environment and help you zero in on subject areas where you need further work.

Review Regularly

Learning is most successful when new information is transferred from working memory to long-term storage on a regular basis. Even if you think you've mastered the subject matter, it's a good idea to review it on a regular basis.

Take Care of Your Physical Health

The state of one's health has a major bearing on one's mental capabilities. Make sure you're getting enough shut-eye, eating right, and being active. Keep your sugar and caffeine intake in check to prevent energy lows.

Develop a Positive Mindset

Keep a good outlook when you're studying. Instead of seeing difficulties as threats, try to see them as chances for personal development. Keeping a positive outlook may do wonders for your drive and toughness.

Use Relaxation Techniques

Learning and memory can be hampered by stress. If you're having trouble dealing with stress, try some relaxation techniques like deep breathing, progressive muscle relaxation, or meditation.

Seek Help When Needed

Don't be afraid to ask for clarification if you're having trouble understanding something. A class, tutor, or study group are all viable options.

Review and Reflect

Spend some time after each study session thinking about what you studied and how well you retained it. This might serve to both reinforce the subject and highlight any gaps in understanding.

Reward Yourself

Use little prizes as motivation. This could be a reward in the form of time off to do something you enjoy or a small token of appreciation.

There is more to effective studying than just putting in extra time. This can be accomplished with some forethought, self-control, and knowledge of your own learning style. You may improve your study habits, test scores, and overall performance with the help of these techniques.

Chapter 2

The Phlebotomy Professional

A phlebotomist is a highly trained healthcare professional who collects blood samples from patients for use in diagnostic procedures, transfusions, scientific studies, and blood donations. In this section, we'll discuss the phlebotomist's job, the qualities they should have as a professional, and the ethical and legal issues that should shape their work.

We go into the technical abilities, attention to detail, interpersonal skills, and in-depth knowledge of safety and hygiene regulations that identify a competent phlebotomist. When dealing with patients, completing paperwork, or conducting experiments, a phlebotomist must always maintain an air of professionalism.

The legal and moral implications of drawing blood are discussed in further depth in this chapter. Tort Law, which deals with civil wrongs that result in harm to others, and Malpractice, which concerns the negligence or incompetence of a professional, are both discussed. Phlebotomists must work within the law and have a firm grasp of these concepts to protect themselves and their employers from liability.

This chapter also discusses risk management in phlebotomy, which is an important but often overlooked topic. Methods for detecting, evaluating, and managing risks to patients, facilities, and phlebotomists' professional reputations are spelled out.

We also explain the Health Insurance Portability and Accountability Act (HIPAA), a federal statute that mandated the development of national standards to prevent the unauthorized disclosure of personal health information. Phlebotomists must be aware of and compliant with HIPAA rules because of the sensitive nature of the patient information they handle.

Last but not least, this section discusses the operational regulatory criteria that direct phlebotomy.

Phlebotomists' adherence to these guidelines ensures that patients continue to receive high-quality, safe, and effective care.

You will finish this chapter with a thorough comprehension of a phlebotomist's job description, duties, and character attributes. You will also learn the basics of the law and ethics as they pertain to phlebotomy, giving you the tools you need to move forward in your career with self-assurance, skill, and integrity.

The Phlebotomist

Phlebotomists are medical staff members who have undergone extensive training in the safe and sanitary collection of blood from patients and donors. They may also work in non-traditional healthcare venues such as outpatient clinics or private homes to provide primary care to patients.

Because most clinical choices are based on laboratory test results, phlebotomists play a crucial role in the diagnosis and treatment of medical diseases. They are also essential in the collection of blood for transfusions for sick patients, which they perform by interviewing donors.

Roles of the Phlebotomist

Patient Identification

Before any blood is drawn from the patient, the phlebotomist needs to ensure that they have an accurate identification of the patient. In most cases, this entails looking at the identifying band that the patient is wearing and comparing it to the information on the laboratory requisition form.

Preparation

The phlebotomist will get the patient ready for the procedure by walking them through it, making sure they are comfortable, and explaining what will happen. They also prepare the necessary equipment for the process, such as needles, devices for collecting blood, tourniquets, and alcohol wipes.

Blood Collection

The collection of blood samples is the primary responsibility of a phlebotomist. Finding a vein that is suitable for the procedure, disinfecting the area, and then inserting a needle to take blood are the basic steps involved. Phlebotomists are required to adhere to standard operating procedures to protect their patients and maximize their level of comfort.

Specimen Handling and Processing

After the collection is complete, the phlebotomist will correctly label the blood samples before delivering them to the laboratory so they may be analyzed. When drawing blood from a patient, the phlebotomist may also be responsible for doing some basic processing on the sample, such as isolating plasma and serum from the entire blood.

Documentation

Phlebotomists are the ones who are accountable for ensuring that patient records are accurate. They keep a record of information such as the time of the blood draw, the amount of blood that is extracted, and any complications or adverse reactions that occur throughout the process.

Patient Interaction

Because they contact directly with patients, phlebotomists frequently take on the role as the "face" of the laboratory. They need to communicate clearly with patients, empathize with them, and reassure them, particularly when dealing with patients who may be nervous about having their blood drawn.

Safety and Compliance

Phlebotomists are responsible for ensuring that all safety requirements are followed in order to stop the transmission of bloodborne diseases. This includes the use of personal protective equipment, the disposal of used needles in an appropriate manner, and the maintenance of a clean and sanitary working environment. In addition to this, they are responsible for adhering to the laws and regulations that govern the privacy and confidentiality of patients.

Quality Control

Phlebotomists play an important part in the quality control processes of laboratories by ensuring the correct collection, storage, and transportation of samples. In addition to this, they are required to take part in quality assurance activities such as tests of their proficiency and ongoing education.

Phlebotomists are responsible for more than merely taking blood samples from patients. They play a vital role in patient care, laboratory procedures, and the delivery of healthcare in general. The responsibilities of the phlebotomist involve technical expertise, abilities related to providing care to patients, attention to detail, and a solid awareness of the standards governing safety and compliance. Because of their varied responsibilities, phlebotomists are an extremely valuable part of the healthcare team.

Professional Traits of the Phlebotomist

Because of the many facets of their job, phlebotomists need to possess a particular set of professional characteristics. Phlebotomists that possess these characteristics are able to properly carry out their responsibilities while maintaining a high level of care and safety for their patients.

Technical Skills

Phlebotomists are required to have a strong command of the technical abilities involved in the process of blood collection. These skills include the selection of veins, the insertion of needles, and the proper processing of blood samples. In addition to this, they need to be proficient in the use of a variety of medical equipment and supplies, such as syringes, vacutainers, and lancets. It is impossible to perform a good and painless venipuncture without a high level of hand-eye coordination as well as dexterity.

Attention to Detail

Phlebotomists are responsible for correctly labeling and storing blood samples to reduce the risk of errors and contamination. When carrying out procedures, documenting information, and adhering to safety laws, they are required to adhere to a stringent set of norms and standards. Any momentary lack in focus can result in major mistakes, which may have an effect on how patients are cared for.

Interpersonal Skills

Because phlebotomists are the only medical professionals that come into close contact with patients, it is essential for them to have strong communication and interpersonal skills. They should be able to properly explain the processes, answer the patient's queries, and calm any fears or anxieties that the patient may have. When it comes to providing a great experience for patients, having empathy, patience, and a friendly approach may go a long way.

Professionalism

In all aspects of healthcare, professionalism is absolutely necessary. Phlebotomists are expected to behave themselves in an ethical manner, which includes protecting the privacy of patients and acting with honesty. They need to show that they are committed to their role by accepting responsibility for their actions and actively exploring opportunities for continual development and learning.

Physical Stamina

Phlebotomy can be a physically taxing profession at times. Phlebotomists are frequently required to work lengthy shifts, spend a significant amount of time on their feet, and occasionally lift or transport patients as well as large pieces of equipment. Therefore, having a robust physical health and a high level of endurance are essential characteristics.

Adaptability

Phlebotomists are required to modify their methods in response to the unique characteristics of each individual patient they serve. It's possible that some people have veins that are difficult to access, while others may be afraid of needles. A phlebotomist must be able to think on their feet and adjust to a variety of different scenarios in order to be successful in their job.

Problem-Solving Skills

Phlebotomists frequently face high-stakes situations in which they must make snap judgments. Phlebotomists are required to make snap decisions regarding how to proceed in the event that a patient experiences an adverse reaction during a blood draw or if a vein is difficult to detect.

Organization Skills

Phlebotomists are responsible for a variety of activities, including managing a full schedule of patients and maintaining accurate records of a large number of blood samples. They are responsible for ensuring that all of the duties are finished in an exact and timely manner, thus they need to have strong organizing abilities.

Stress Management

The environments in which healthcare is provided can be tense and frenetic at times. Phlebotomists need to be able to successfully manage their stress in order to keep their performance at a high level and give the best possible treatment for their patients.

Knowledgeable

Phlebotomists are required to have a strong awareness of the procedures involved in venipuncture, as well as the protocols for maintaining patient safety. They should also keep themselves apprised of the most recent breakthroughs in their respective fields.

Compassion

Dealing with patients who could be nervous or in pain is a common part of a phlebotomist's job. When it comes to giving these patients with assistance and comfort, compassion and empathy are absolutely necessary.

Integrity

Since phlebotomists deal with confidential health information, they are expected to maintain a high level of honesty and ethical conduct. They have a responsibility to protect the privacy of their patients and adhere to all of their profession's ethical and legal requirements.

Phlebotomists that are effective possess a balance of technical and interpersonal abilities, as well as professionalism, adaptability, and a dedication to the care and protection of their patients.

Legal and Ethical Considerations

Phlebotomy is governed by a set of legal and ethical issues that safeguard the safety, dignity, and rights of patients. These factors can be found in the Phlebotomy Practice Act. Phlebotomists should adhere to these guiding principles in all aspects of their professional behavior, including decision-making.

Consent

A patient is required to provide their informed consent prior to having blood drawn from them by a phlebotomist. This indicates that the patient has been given an explanation of the process by the phlebotomist, including its purpose as well as any possible hazards, and that they have accepted to have the operation performed. The law requires that consent be given, and if it is not given, a person may be accused of battery or assault if the procedure is carried out.

Confidentiality and Privacy

Phlebotomists have a legal responsibility to protect the privacy of their patients' medical records in accordance with the Health Insurance Portability and Accountability Act (HIPAA). They are not permitted to reveal test results, patient names, or any other identifiable information to any individual who is not directly involved in the care of the patient. Any violation of a patient's right to privacy can result in severe repercussions, both professionally and legally.

Professional Competence

To practice as a phlebotomist in the United States, one must be able to legally establish a particular degree of professional competence. This indicates that they need to have the appropriate training, abilities, and certification in order to carry out their responsibilities in a manner that is both safe and successful. If a phlebotomist engages in activities that are beyond the scope of their practice or carries out a procedure for which they do not have the necessary skills, they may be subject to legal action for carelessness or malpractice.

Duty of Care

Phlebotomists have a responsibility to provide high-quality care to their patients. Because of this, they are obligated to put up their maximum effort to protect the health and safety of the patients under their care. This involves adhering to all safety regulations, utilizing sterile equipment, and taking the proper steps in the event that a patient experiences an adverse response while having blood drawn from them.

Ethical Considerations

Phlebotomists are also required to abide by a code of ethics in their line of work. These include treating patients with dignity and autonomy, acting in the patients' best interests, and being honest and transparent in their interactions with patients and other healthcare professionals. Respecting the dignity and autonomy of patients is just one of these.

When practicing phlebotomy, it is imperative to keep legal and ethical concerns in mind at all times. Phlebotomists are held to these standards so that their professional behavior is consistent with the protection of patients' rights and well-being. Phlebotomists can ensure that they deliver the greatest degree of care to their patients while also safeguarding themselves from the possibility of legal ramifications if they adhere to these rules and follow them to the letter.

Tort Law

In the context of phlebotomy, the concept of tort law refers to civil wrongs that end up causing the patient to suffer injury. These might be deliberate acts like violence, or they can be careless omissions like neglect. Phlebotomists are required to be familiar with these rules and to behave themselves in a manner that reduces the likelihood of their patients being injured.

Malpractice

When a healthcare worker, such as a phlebotomist, causes injury to a patient as a result of their negligence or incompetence, this is considered to be medical malpractice. Some examples of this might be neglecting to follow the appropriate procedures, wrongly labeling blood samples, or inflicting unneeded damage while drawing blood from a patient.

Risk Management

The process of recognizing possible dangers and devising countermeasures is an essential part of risk management. In the field of phlebotomy, this may entail performing routine checks on the equipment, according to the established safety procedures, and ensuring that the working space is kept clean and sanitary.

Health Insurance Portability and Accountability Act (HIPAA)

The Health Insurance Portability and Accountability Act of 1996 (HIPAA) is a piece of legislation that was passed into law at the federal level in the United States. It was intended to alleviate constraints on healthcare insurance coverage, modernize the flow of healthcare information, and establish how personally identifiable information that is stored by the healthcare and healthcare insurance businesses should be protected against fraud and theft.

Overview of HIPAA

The major purpose of the Health Insurance Portability and Accountability Act of 1996 (HIPAA) is to simplify the process by which individuals can maintain their health insurance coverage, to preserve the privacy and integrity of patients' medical information, and to assist the healthcare industry in better managing its administrative expenses. Fundamentally, it ensures that individuals can take their health insurance coverage with them from one employment to another and it imposes security standards to protect the confidentiality of healthcare information.

The Privacy Rule (the Rule)

The HIPAA Privacy Rule is an essential part of the Health Insurance Portability and Accountability Act (HIPAA), which sets national standards for the protection of individuals' medical records and other personal health information. It is applicable to health plans, healthcare clearinghouses, as well as healthcare providers, who carry out various transactions related to healthcare electronically.

It is required under the Rule that sufficient protections be in place to preserve the privacy of personal health information, and it establishes limits and conditions on the uses and disclosures that may be made of such information without the authorization of the patient. The Rule also provides patients with rights over their health information, including the rights to inspect and acquire a copy of their medical records, as well as the right to request that any errors in those data be corrected.

The Security Rule

The HIPAA Security Rule is yet another essential component of this law. This rule addresses Electronic Protected Health Information, or ePHI for short. It is intended to supplement the Privacy Rule. It establishes national guidelines for the protection of patient information that is either electronically stored or transferred. To comply with HIPAA's Security Rule, covered entities must keep reasonable and necessary administrative, technical, and physical measures in place to protect electronic protected health information (ePHI).

Specifically, covered entities must

Ensure the privacy, security, and availability of any and all electronic protected health information (ePHI) that they generate, receive, store, or transfer.

Determine which dangers to the information's security or integrity can be reasonably anticipated and take measures to guard against those threats.

Protect against uses or disclosures that are not permitted, even if they can be fairly expected.

Ensure that their workforce complies with the regulations.

Impact on Phlebotomy

Phlebotomists are considered to be a part of the healthcare provider industry and are therefore required to comply with HIPAA rules. They are obligated to handle patient information discretely while also ensuring that it is stored and delivered in a secure manner. This encompasses anything and everything related to a patient's health, including verbal communication, written records, and computerized data.

Phlebotomists have a duty of care to ensure that they do not disclose private patient information in public spaces, that they do not lose track of patient records, and that they do not transmit patient information over unsecure digital channels. If you do not comply with these regulations, there may be disciplinary action taken against you, as well as significant fines and even serious legal implications.

Patient Rights under HIPAA

Under the Health Insurance Portability and Accountability Act (HIPAA), patients have certain rights, including the right to access their own medical information, the right to ask for modifications to their records, the right to get notice of how their information may be used, and the right to choose whether or not to share their information with others. If they believe that their rights have been infringed, they also have the right to register a complaint with the Department of Health and Human Services or with the healthcare provider that they currently use.

The Health Insurance Portability and Accountability Act (HIPAA) is vital legislation that protects patient health information, preserves patients' rights, and directs medical personnel, such as phlebotomists, on how to handle patient data in a responsible manner. It is essential for everyone involved in patient care to have a solid awareness of the HIPAA standards and to comply with them.

Operational Regulatory Standards

In the context of phlebotomy, the term "operational regulatory standards" refers to the rules and guidelines that control the procedures, methods, and behavior that take place inside a phlebotomy environment. Phlebotomy services are intended to be safe, accurate, and of high quality, thus these criteria have been established by various regulatory agencies and are intended to be followed.

Clinical and Laboratory Standards Institute (CLSI)

Phlebotomy is one of the clinical testing disciplines that is regulated and governed by the Clinical Laboratory Standards Institute (CLSI). These standards address a variety of facets of the blood collection process, including the protocols for venipuncture and capillary puncture, the order of draw, and patient identification.

Occupational Safety and Health Administration (OSHA)

Phlebotomy is governed by a number of OSHA regulations and guidelines. These include regulations on bloodborne pathogens, which address exposure management strategies, the use of personal protective equipment (PPE), and procedures for dealing with exposure occurrences. Specifically, these regulations concern bloodborne pathogens. Other OSHA rules that are pertinent to phlebotomy include those on ergonomics, recording of work-related injuries and illnesses, and hazard communication. Hazardous compounds utilized in the laboratory are the subject of the hazard communication standards.

Centers for Disease Control and Prevention (CDC)

The Centers for Disease prevention and Prevention (CDC) offers standards for infection prevention in healthcare settings. These rules are essential in phlebotomy. These standards address a wide range of topics, including proper hand hygiene, the use of personal protective equipment (PPE), and the cleaning of equipment and surfaces. The Centers for Disease Control and Prevention (CDC) also offers guidelines for dealing with particular infectious agents that might be found in a phlebotomy setting.

Food and Drug Administration (FDA)

The Food and Drug Administration (FDA) is in charge of regulating the production and sale of phlebotomy-related medical devices, such as needles, lancets, and blood collection tubes. They make sure that the products they sell are risk-free and effective, and that the production techniques they use are up to par with quality requirements.

Joint Commission

Accreditation for medical facilities, such as hospitals and outpatient clinics, can be obtained through the Joint Commission. Among the facilities that can receive accreditation are those that offer phlebotomy services. To get and keep this certification, a business must demonstrate that it satisfies the Commission's requirements pertaining to both quality and safety. These standards cover a wide range of topics, including patient rights, infection control, the administration of medical equipment, and the credentials of staff members and their training.

Health Insurance Portability and Accountability Act (HIPAA)

Phlebotomists are required to comply with the HIPAA's privacy and security regulations in order to legally collect, use, disclose, and maintain patients' health information. Phlebotomists are required to comply with the HIPAA regulations on patient identification, the completion of test requisition forms, and any and all discussions with patient information.

State and Local Regulations

Phlebotomy operations may be subject to rules imposed by their respective states as well as by their respective municipalities, in addition to those imposed by the federal government. The accreditation of phlebotomists, the licensing of laboratories, and the proper disposal of medical waste may be among these requirements.

It is absolutely necessary to comply with these operational regulatory standards in order to guarantee the high quality and personal safety of phlebotomy services. It aids in the prevention of errors and mishaps, shields patients and staff from injury, and helps the phlebotomy profession preserve its integrity and reputation. Phlebotomists and the businesses that hire them need to be aware of these criteria in order to adopt the necessary processes and receive the necessary training.

Chapter 3

Safety Protocols and Compliance

The third chapter of this manual looks into the essentials of phlebotomy safety measures and regulatory compliance. Maintaining a secure facility is crucial for the well-being of both patients and medical staff. This not only guarantees that patients receive high-quality care, but it also maintains the confidence and trustworthiness of the healthcare industry as a whole.

We begin our examination of safety regulations and standards with those designed to keep workers and patients safe in the workplace. We will also examine operational standards rules that control the methods used in a phlebotomy setting to ensure patient safety and the highest level of care.

Protecting patients' health information in accordance with the Health Insurance Portability and Accountability Act (HIPAA) is a vital aspect of the safety standards. We will also talk about the ethical principles that all medical personnel, including phlebotomists, should follow.

For precise diagnosis and treatment, quality control of laboratory equipment is crucial. The steps taken to guarantee that phlebotomy equipment is up to par for safe and efficient use will be scrutinized.

We will also discuss transmission-based and universal precautions for limiting the spread of disease. Controlling exposure, properly disposing of biohazards and sharps, and other aseptic and infection-prevention procedures will also be covered.

Clinical Laboratory Improvement Amendments (CLIA) waived tests, which are less complex and can be used in a wider range of healthcare settings, will also be discussed in this chapter.

Infection control relies heavily on regular hand washing. We'll talk about why and how hand cleanliness is so crucial in a phlebotomy scenario.

Since medical problems can arise at any time in a clinical setting, we will also go over the importance of phlebotomists having CPR and first aid training.

Finally, we will discuss the importance of record-keeping and reporting for continuing security and conformity. Care for patients can be transparent and accountable only if proper documentation is kept.

This chapter will equip readers with in-depth information on phlebotomy safety protocols and compliance, which is critical for the health and safety of both patients and medical staff.

Workplace Safety Regulations

In healthcare settings, numerous regulatory agencies implement workplace safety laws with the overarching goal of protecting the health and safety of both staff and patients. Phlebotomy-specific rules span numerous domains, including as workplace security, infection prevention, equipment care, and the proper disposal of potentially dangerous substances.

Occupational Safety and Health Administration (OSHA)

When it comes to workplace safety in the United States, OSHA is the go-to government agency for rulemaking and enforcement. The Bloodborne infections Standard is a crucial OSHA rule for phlebotomists since it details how to prevent occupational exposure to bloodborne infections. Safe needle handling and disposal, as well as the use of PPE and exposure management plans, are all required by the rules.

General Safety

Phlebotomy-specific legislation for the workplace address a wide range of environmental factors. Keeping the building clean, clearing away clutter, installing sufficient lighting, and routinely disinfecting all surfaces are all important measures to take to reduce the risk of the spread of disease.

Ergonomics

Ergonomic problems are common among phlebotomists due to the repeated nature of their work. Ergonomic factors, such as chair and table height, excellent body mechanics throughout processes, and regular breaks to minimize repetitive strain injuries, are therefore also addressed by workplace safety rules.

Hazard Communication

Another important safety rule is OSHA's Hazard Communication Standard (HCS). It's the employer's responsibility to educate workers on the risks posed by chemicals used in the workplace. Phlebotomists may be exposed to lab chemicals like disinfectants and reagents while performing their duties.

Equipment Safety

Use, maintenance, and disposal of equipment are all aspects of safety that must be addressed by law. Needles, syringes, and tourniquets are just some of the tools that phlebotomists need to be proficient with. It is important to notify and repair any broken or malfunctioning equipment on a regular basis.

Handling and Disposal of Biohazardous Waste

Biohazardous waste, such as used needles, blood-soaked gauze, and other contaminated items, must be handled and disposed of correctly to prevent any potential safety issues. Puncture-resistant sharps containers and biohazard bags or containers with labels are required under OSHA regulations.

Fire and Emergency Safety

Fire and other emergency measures are also covered by workplace safety standards. This entails doing things like holding regular drills for emergency evacuation and making sure all exits are easily accessible at all times and that fire extinguishers are in good working order.

Training and Compliance

Regular training and education is necessary for compliance with safety laws. Phlebotomists should receive ongoing training in modern best practices for patient protection. Training doesn't end after the first day; new tools, processes, or rules may necessitate more sessions.

The phlebotomy profession relies heavily on compliance with workplace safety rules. They make it so that phlebotomists can do their jobs without putting themselves or patients in danger. These guidelines serve as an industry standard against which care quality and conduct can be measured.

Operational Standards Regulations

The purpose of phlebotomy quality, safety, and accuracy regulations established by operational standards. All three levels of government (federal, state, and local) have their own sets of regulations outlining and enforcing these.

Important criteria for operations include:

Clinical and Laboratory Standards Institute (CLSI)

They outline standards for phlebotomy and other forms of clinical testing. Patients must be identified, the order in which blood is drawn, and the protocols for venipuncture and capillary puncture must be followed. Guidelines for the care, transportation, and storage of specimens are also included.

The Joint Commission

Phlebotomy services are included in the scope of healthcare providers that they accredit. Patient rights, infection control, medical equipment management, and staff qualifications and training are just a few of the quality and safety standards that must be met in order to obtain and keep this accreditation.

State and Local Regulations

Phlebotomist certification, laboratory accreditation, and the proper disposal of medical waste are all topics that could be subject to further state restrictions.

HIPAA Regulations

Patient medical records are shielded from prying eyes by HIPAA, the Health Insurance Portability and Accountability Act. Phlebotomists are subject to many HIPAA rules:

Privacy Rule

The Privacy Rule mandates the confidentiality of patients' medical records. Phlebotomists are responsible for maintaining the privacy of their patients' information on all test labels, computer systems, and requisition forms. To prevent accidental disclosure, all conversations involving patient data must take place in private.

Security Rule

Electronic PHI (ePHI) is under the purview of the Security Rule. Phlebotomists are responsible for maintaining the confidentiality of patient data and must adhere to strict rules while accessing medical records electronically.

Breach Notification Rule

In the event of a breach of unencrypted PHI, the Breach Notification Rule specifies what must be done. In some situations, the media and the Secretary of Health and Human Services may also need to be notified.

Enforcement Rule

The penalties for violating HIPAA rules are outlined in the Enforcement Rule. Both phlebotomists and their employers risk heavy fines for violations of these regulations.

Phlebotomy is a field that relies heavily on compliance with operational standards laws and HIPAA rules. The quality and safety of phlebotomy processes are governed by operational standards rules, while patient privacy is safeguarded by HIPAA laws. A phlebotomist's ability to comprehend and adhere to these rules is crucial to the success of the profession.

Ethical Standards

Phlebotomy ethics are of the utmost importance when it comes to giving patients with care that is both caring and considerate. The following is a list of the ethical considerations that apply to phlebotomy:

Respect for Autonomy

Patients have the responsibility and the right to make educated decisions regarding their own medical care. Before beginning any procedure, phlebotomists are required to get the patient's informed consent, during which they will go over the process, the risks involved, and the potential benefits.

Beneficence and Nonmaleficence

Phlebotomists are obligated to put the patient's welfare first and work to prevent any potential injury. This includes carrying out procedures skillfully, reducing the amount of discomfort experienced by patients, and strictly adhering to all safety measures.

Justice

Patients should be handled in a manner that is equitable and free from discrimination. Patients of any age, gender, or ethnicity are entitled to the same level of care, regardless of any other considerations that may come into play.

Confidentiality

Phlebotomists are obligated to protect the privacy and confidentiality of their patients. This includes acting in accordance with the HIPAA requirements and taking precautions to prevent the disclosure of patient information without the required consent.

Professionalism

Phlebotomists are required to uphold professional standards, which include presenting themselves in a manner befitting their profession, communicating in a manner that is polite and effective, and acting with integrity in all that they do.

Lab Equipment Quality Control

In a phlebotomy setting, quality control makes certain that all of the equipment and supplies are operating as they should, which helps to ensure that test results are accurate and trustworthy. The following are some of the most important aspects:

Equipment Maintenance

It is helpful to do routine maintenance on machinery, such as centrifuges, in accordance with the instructions provided by the manufacturer. This helps to ensure that the machinery will continue to function properly and will last as long as possible.

Regular Calibration

To guarantee that they are producing accurate readings, measuring devices like centrifuges and glucose meters need to have their accuracy checked on a regular basis.

Proper Storage

Phlebotomy equipment, such as evacuated tubes, has specific storage requirements that must be met in order to preserve its integrity. This includes storage in a controlled temperature environment as well as protection from light where appropriate.

Expiration Dates

There is a time limit on the use of any and all supplies, including the blood collection tubes and chemicals. Supplies that have expired can introduce errors into test findings and should never be used.

Quality Control Logs

Phlebotomy facilities ought to keep quality control records, in which they should document the upkeep and calibration of their equipment, as well as any problems or peculiarities that may arise. This makes it possible to monitor the functioning of the equipment over time and to spot any difficulties that keep cropping up.

Troubleshooting

Phlebotomists ought to receive training in the fundamentals of equipment maintenance and repair. In the event that a problem cannot be fixed, they should be aware of whom to speak to in order to receive additional support.

The practice of phlebotomy requires strict adherence to ethical norms as well as quality control measures for laboratory equipment. Phlebotomists are held to ethical standards in order to ensure that the treatment they provide to patients is of the highest possible standard. Quality control ensures that phlebotomy processes and test results are accurate and reliable.

Standard Precautions

In healthcare settings, standard precautions are a collection of infection control procedures that are aimed to reduce the risk of spreading infectious pathogens to patients. These safety measures need to be implemented for each and every patient, irrespective of whether an infection has been positively identified or not. The following are important aspects of standard precautions:

Hand Hygiene

It is essential to practice correct hand hygiene in order to stop the transmission of illnesses. Before and after having contact with each patient, phlebotomists should wash their hands thoroughly with soap and water or apply an alcohol-based hand sanitizer to their hands.

Personal Protective Equipment (PPE)

When there is a potential for exposure to blood, other bodily fluids, or other potentially infectious materials, it is imperative that personal protective equipment (PPE) be worn. Examples of PPE include gloves, gowns, masks, and eye protection. Phlebotomists are required to wear personal protective equipment that is suitable for the treatments they are performing and the risk of exposure.

Respiratory Hygiene and Cough Etiquette

Phlebotomists should urge patients to cover their mouth and nose when coughing or sneezing, give tissues and no-touch receptacles for disposal, and practice good respiratory hygiene themselves. Patients should be encouraged to cover their mouth and nose when coughing or sneezing.

Safe Injection Practices

Phlebotomists are required to adhere to safe injection practices, which include using a new needle and syringe for each patient, preventing the reuse of single-use vials, and making sure that sharps are disposed of in the appropriate manner.

Safe Handling of Contaminated Equipment and Surfaces

The proper cleaning and disinfecting procedures should be carried out on all contaminated pieces of equipment and surfaces. Phlebotomists are expected to follow the protocols that have been developed for the cleaning and disinfection of equipment between each encounter with a patient.

Transmission-Based Precautions

Transmission-based precautions are supplementary infection control measures that are used for patients with known or suspected infections who require additional precautions over and beyond normal precautions. These patients are given transmission-based precautions. There are three distinct categories of preventative measures that are based on transmission:

Contact Precautions

Patients who are known to have or who may have infections that can be passed on to others through direct or indirect contact should follow these safety measures. When entering a patient's room, phlebotomists are required to don gowns and gloves, and they must adhere to strict regulations regarding the cleaning and disinfection of equipment and the surrounding environment.

Droplet Precautions

Patients who are known to have or who are suspected of having infections that can be spread by respiratory droplets are given droplet precautions. Phlebotomists are required to observe proper procedures for respiratory hygiene and should always protect themselves while working in close proximity to patients by using protective eyewear and masks.

Airborne Precautions

Patients with known or suspected diseases that are spread by minute particles that remain suspended in the air for extended periods of time are given special instructions to follow called airborne precautions. When entering a patient's room, phlebotomists are required to don a respirator (such as a N95 mask) and adhere to a predetermined set of protocols in order to prevent the spread of airborne diseases.

Phlebotomists need to be aware of the particular safety measures that must be taken for each type of infection, and they must adhere to the procedures that have been developed in order to stop the transmission of infectious agents.

When it comes to limiting the spread of illnesses in hospital settings, the use of both standard precautions and transmission-based precautions are absolutely essential. Phlebotomists are responsible for adhering to these measures, performing appropriate hand hygiene, using suitable personal protective equipment, and following specific protocols dependent on the infection state of the patient in order to protect both the patients and the healthcare professionals.

Exposure Control

Exposure control is a term that refers to the procedures that are taken to minimize the danger of exposure to infectious materials, such as bloodborne pathogens, for those who work in the healthcare industry. This includes phlebotomists. The following are important factors of exposure control:

Engineering Controls

Engineering controls are physical or mechanical devices that are designed to isolating the hazard or eliminating it entirely. Engineering controls in the field of phlebotomy include things like sharps containers, safety-engineered devices (such needleless systems or safety needles), and biohazard spill kits. These safeguards help reduce the possibility of unintentional needlesticks or other forms of contamination with blood-borne infections.

Controls over Work Practices

Controls used in the workplace, also known as work practice controls, are procedures and practices that lessen the likelihood of being exposed. Work practice controls for phlebotomists include maintaining appropriate hand hygiene, adhering to safe injection techniques, avoiding the recapping of needles, and correctly storing and disposing of contaminated materials.

Personal Protective Equipment (PPE)

Personal protective equipment is an integral part of exposure control. Phlebotomists are required to use the proper personal protective equipment (PPE), which includes gloves, gowns, masks, and eye protection, in order to protect themselves from the risk of being exposed to blood or other potentially infectious materials. To reduce the likelihood of becoming contaminated, personal protective equipment (PPE) should be worn continuously and removed in the correct manner.

Post-Exposure Evaluation and Follow-up

It is important for phlebotomists to have access to post-exposure evaluation and follow-up protocols in the event that an exposure occurrence occurs. This involves notifying the proper authorities, obtaining an appropriate medical evaluation, and adhering to any post-exposure prophylaxis or therapy that may be required.

Disposal of Biohazards and Sharps

In order to prevent injuries, exposure to pathogens, and the spread of illnesses, it is essential to dispose of biohazards and sharps in the appropriate manner. Here are some important factors to take into account:

Sharps Disposal

Needles, lancets, and any other sharp objects that have been used should be disposed of as soon as possible in puncture-resistant containers, which are also often known as "sharps containers."

These containers must to be placed in a convenient location, adjacent to the area where they will be utilized, and clearly labeled. After they have been used up, sharps containers need to be sealed and disposed of in accordance with the rules and regulations that govern the area.

Biohazard Waste Disposal

Other types of biohazardous trash, such as blood-soaked gauze, bandages, or cultures, should be disposed of in bags or containers specifically designed for biohazardous waste. These bags need to be airtight, labelled with a biohazard emblem, and disposed of in accordance with the rules that are in place in the area.

Segregation and Storage

It is imperative that biohazardous waste and sharps be properly compartmentalized and stored in order to eliminate the risk of inadvertent exposure and contamination. It is possible to avoid the spread of germs by separating biohazardous waste from other types of trash and by ensuring that correct storage conditions, including temperature control, are maintained.

Transportation and Disposal

It is imperative that the biohazardous waste and sharps be transported from the healthcare facility to the approved disposal facility in accordance with all of the relevant local legislation and protocols. Collaboration with waste management organizations that are experts in the secure transportation and disposal of biohazardous materials is frequently required as part of this process.

To ensure the proper and safe disposal of biohazards and sharps, phlebotomists should get training on proper disposal techniques, be conversant with local regulations, and follow established protocols.

Controlling the exposure to infections and ensuring that sharps and biohazards are disposed of properly are two of the most important things that can be done to protect healthcare personnel, such as phlebotomists, from the risk of injury and contamination. Maintaining a safe working environment requires a strict adherence to engineering controls, work practice controls, the appropriate use of personal protective equipment (PPE), and the following of appropriate disposal policy.

CLIA Waived Tests

CLIA (Clinical Laboratory Improvement Amendments) waived tests are a group of laboratory tests that are regarded to have a low risk of error. These tests are exempt from the CLIA (Clinical Laboratory Improvement Amendments). The Food and Drug Administration (FDA) of the United States has given its stamp of approval to these tests on the grounds that they are straightforward to use and, when carried out appropriately, generate reliable findings. The following are some important considerations with reference to CLIA waived tests:

Definition

CLIA waived tests are typically point-of-care tests that can be conducted in locations other than a conventional laboratory, such as in a doctor's office, clinic, or pharmacy. These locations are exempt from the CLIA's testing requirements. They are given the status of "waived" because the FDA has determined that even if they are carried out improperly, they do not provide any kind of major risk.

Examples of CLIA Waived Tests

The Clinical Laboratory Improvement Amendments of 1988 (CLIA) exempted certain fast strep tests, pregnancy tests, urine dipsticks, and glucose meters for the purpose of monitoring blood glucose levels. These examinations are often developed to be simple in both their usage and their interpretation, with a low potential for making mistakes.

Training and Competency

Even since CLIA waived tests are thought to have a minimal risk of error, it is still extremely important for phlebotomists and other medical professionals to get the proper training and demonstrate that they are competent in order to perform these tests. Training may be offered either directly by the manufacturer or indirectly through specialized educational programs.

Quality Control

Even if there is a decreased potential for error with CLIA waived testing, quality control procedures still need to be adhered to in order to guarantee accurate and trustworthy results. This involves ensuring that any testing equipment is appropriately calibrated on a regular basis, adhering to any quality control protocols that are provided by the manufacturer, and correctly documenting any test findings.

Regulatory Compliance

Facilities that perform CLIA waived tests are required to comply with all applicable regulatory standards, such as maintaining the appropriate documentation and reporting. The accuracy and dependability of test findings are improved when laboratories comply with the regulations set forth by the CLIA.

Aseptic and Infection Control

Phlebotomy is a field that requires meticulous attention to detail about aseptic technique and infection control in order to forestall the spread of infectious pathogens and preserve a sterile atmosphere. Among the most important considerations are:

Hand Hygiene

Before and after contact with each individual patient, it is vital to practice correct hand hygiene. This involves either washing one's hands with soap and water or using a hand sanitizer that contains alcohol. This helps to reduce the likelihood of illnesses being passed from person to person as well as the possibility of cross-contamination.

Personal Protective Equipment (PPE)

It is essential to protect the phlebotomist as well as the patient by wearing the proper personal protective equipment (PPE), which may include gloves, masks, gowns, and eye protection. In order to stop the spread of infectious pathogens, personal protective equipment (PPE) must be worn at all times and removed in the correct manner.

Aseptic Technique

When performing venipuncture or any other type of invasive procedure, phlebotomists are required to use aseptic technique. This includes properly disinfecting the place where the venipuncture will be performed, using sterile gloves, and utilizing sterile equipment for each individual patient in order to prevent the spread of germs.

Handling and Disposal of Contaminated Materials

Materials that have been contaminated, such as worn gloves, gauze, or other throwaway items, need to be disposed of in approved biohazard containers in accordance with the guidelines that have been developed. This stops the transmission of infectious pathogens and ensures that potentially hazardous products are handled and disposed of correctly.

Environmental Cleaning

A clean and sterile atmosphere can be maintained with the help of routine cleaning and disinfection of work areas, as well as surfaces, equipment, and other locations. This involves making use of the proper disinfectants and adhering to the predetermined procedures specified for the frequency and methods of cleaning.

Adherence to Standard and Transmission-Based Precautions

It is essential to practice good hand hygiene, wear personal protective equipment (PPE), and handle sharp objects in a safe manner in order to prevent the spread of infection. In addition, in order to stop the spread of pathogens, it is vital to adhere to certain transmission-based precautions when working with patients who are known to have infections or who may have infections. These precautions can be broken down into three categories: contact, droplet, and airborne.

Hand Hygiene

In a healthcare environment, proper hygiene of the hands is an essential component of infection control and the prevention of the transmission of germs. It is absolutely necessary for phlebotomists to practice good hand hygiene in order to protect not only their patients but also their fellow medical professionals. Here are some crucial points regarding hand hygiene:

Handwashing vs. Hand Sanitizing

Hand hygiene should always begin with washing one's hands with soap and water. This is the most effective strategy for removing dirt, bacteria, and other potentially harmful agents from one's hands. When hands are clearly dirty, before eating, and after using the restroom are the appropriate times to execute this action. Hand sanitizers that include alcohol can be used as a substitute for soap and water in situations where neither of those items is easily available.

Technique for Handwashing

Hands should be moistened with water that is running cleanly, soap should be applied, and hands should be forcefully rubbed together for at least twenty seconds while performing proper handwashing technique. It is important to thoroughly clean the entire surface area of the hands, including the palms, the backs of the hands, the fingers, and the nails. Perform a thorough hand washing followed by drying with a clean towel or an air dryer.

When to Perform Hand Hygiene

Even when gloves are worn, phlebotomists are still responsible for maintaining proper hand hygiene before and after working with each patient. In addition to this, it is also important to practice proper hand hygiene after contacting any surfaces or items in the surrounding area, after removing gloves, and both before and after engaging in invasive procedures.

Nail Care

For proper hand hygiene, it is necessary to keep the nails short, clean, and well-maintained at all times. Pathogens can be harbored under long nails or in nail extensions, putting a person's hand hygiene at risk. It is essential to keep nails clipped and free from nail polish or artificial nails in order to prevent cross-contamination and improper handwashing, both of which can be hampered by either of these factors.

Role of Gloves

Proper hand hygiene is not a suitable replacement for donning gloves when the situation calls for them. When doing phlebotomy procedures, one should always wear gloves to protect against coming into contact with blood or other physiological fluids. However, hand hygiene should still be undertaken before donning gloves and after glove removal to guarantee proper cleanliness.

CPR and First Aid

Phlebotomists are occasionally put in high-pressure circumstances that require them to react quickly and have a thorough understanding of CPR (Cardiopulmonary Resuscitation) and other first aid procedures. Here are some important details regarding cardiopulmonary resuscitation (CPR) and first aid:

CPR

When a person's breathing or heartbeat has stopped, one can perform cardiopulmonary resuscitation (CPR), which is a technique that can save their life. Phlebotomists should be educated in the fundamentals of cardiopulmonary resuscitation (CPR), which includes chest compressions and rescue breathing. During a cardiac arrest, starting chest compressions and ventilations (CPR) as soon as possible can dramatically improve a person's chances of surviving.

First Aid Skills

Having the knowledge and abilities necessary for first aid is essential in order to provide emergency care for acute illnesses or injuries before expert medical assistance comes. Phlebotomists need to be trained to recognize and respond appropriately to a variety of medical crises, including but not limited to: bleeding, burns, allergic reactions, seizures, and fainting. Phlebotomists that have received first aid training are better equipped to stabilize a patient's condition and stop any more damage from occurring.

Certification and Recertification

Training in first aid and CPR normally consists of courses leading to certification, which in turn typically require frequent recertification to ensure that skills are kept current. Phlebotomists should make it a point to keep their certifications up to date and participate in ongoing training and recertification activities in order to ensure they are adequately prepared for any unexpected circumstances.

Emergency Response Planning

The provision of emergency medical equipment and a set of guidelines for how to respond to various types of incidents are both essential components of the emergency response plans that healthcare facilities should have in place. Phlebotomists need to become familiar with these strategies and be aware of their function as well as the responsibilities that fall under their purview in the event of an emergency.

Documentation

The provision of first aid should always include the documentation of any incidents. Phlebotomists have a responsibility to accurately document the specifics of any emergency situation that may arise, including the steps that were taken, the vital signs of the patient, and any communication with emergency medical services.

Documentation and Reporting

Correct documentation and timely reporting are essential for sustaining quality care and protecting patients from harm. Accurately recording and reporting phlebotomy data is crucial to smooth operations and clear communication among medical staff. Important factors to remember while documenting and reporting:

Patient Identification

Documentation relies heavily on correct patient identification. Before drawing blood or taking a patient's vitals, phlebotomists must double-check their identity using at least two different identities. Clear and consistent documentation of this information is required across all applicable records.

Requisition Forms

Phlebotomists need to be thorough while filling up requisition forms, making sure that patient information, test orders, and any relevant notes or instructions are all included. To avoid mistakes and boost processing speed in the lab, legible handwriting or electronic entry is essential.

Test Results

Reporting test results quickly and accurately is essential for patient care. Phlebotomists have the responsibility of ensuring that properly labeled request forms are submitted to the lab for analysis. In addition, they must be diligent in reporting abnormal or critical data and conveying this information to the right healthcare practitioners in accordance with established standards.

Incident Reports

Phebotomists are required to fill out incident reports whenever something untoward happens during phlebotomy procedures, such as a needlestick injury or a patient falling. Time, place, names, and descriptions of those engaged and the events itself can all be found in these reports. Reporting incidents makes it easier to look into what went wrong, figure out why it happened, and take action to prevent it from happening again in the future.

HIPAA Compliance

The privacy and confidentiality of patients must be preserved in accordance with HIPAA guidelines in all documentation. Phlebotomists need to be careful about discussing patients' private information in public, keeping electronic records safe, and adhering to all applicable regulations regarding the use and disclosure of patients' personal health data.

Legal and Regulatory Requirements

Phlebotomists need to understand the documentation and reporting standards mandated by law. This involves knowing how long you have to keep patient records, keeping them safe, and following any local, state, or federal rules that may be in effect.

Key Takeaways of Safety and Compliance

Adherence to Safety Protocols

Safety procedures and guidelines have been developed to prevent the spread of disease from phlebotomists to their patients. Aseptic techniques are adhered to, as well as the use of PPE and clean hands before and during procedures.

Compliance with Operational Standards

Delivery of high-quality, safe, and efficient phlebotomy services is ensured by adhering to operating standards such as those established by CLSI and OSHA. Phlebotomists are obligated to maintain and regularly apply these guidelines.

Awareness of HIPAA Regulations

Protecting patient privacy and confidentiality requires an understanding of, and adherence to, HIPAA regulations. Careful handling of patient health records, obtaining necessary consent, and secure data storage and transmission are all responsibilities of phlebotomists.

Effective Communication and Documentation

Maintaining continuity of care and reducing errors both depend on clear and accurate communication through documentation. Phlebotomists need to be able to communicate with other members of the healthcare team, keep detailed records of their work, and quickly and accurately report test results.

Continuous Education and Training

Phlebotomists must maintain their knowledge of the most recent safety procedures, regulatory standards, and best practices through ongoing education and training. In this way, they can keep up with the field's constant evolution and ensure that their patients always receive the best care possible.

Phlebotomists improve patient care and foster a safety culture by paying close attention to documentation and reporting methods and following all applicable regulations and guidelines.

Chapter 4

The Basics of Human Anatomy

A thorough familiarity with human anatomy is necessary for successful venipuncture and the protection of patients in the field of phlebotomy. This section of the book introduces the reader to the fundamentals of human anatomy, covering such topics as anatomical terminology and the body's primary systems and structures.

Anatomy is the study of the human body as a whole, including its structure and organization. It entails naming and describing many components of the human body. Phlebotomists rely on their knowledge of anatomy to precisely detect veins, grasp the roles of various physiological systems, and make sense of the connections between the structures they encounter during venipuncture.

Important components of human anatomy, such as the locations, orientations, and structures described by anatomical words, will be discussed in this chapter. The next section will examine the body's principal systems, beginning with the skin, hair, and nails that make up the integumentary system. We will go into great depth discussing the skeletal system, the muscular system, the neurological system, the respiratory system, the digestive system, the urinary system, the endocrine system, the reproductive system, and the cardiovascular system.

Since the skin is typically the site of venipuncture, knowledge of the integumentary system is very important for phlebotomists. Understanding the veins' locations and functions, as well as how to reach them during venipuncture, requires knowledge of the skeletal and muscular systems.

The nervous system is extremely important because of the signals it transmits and the functions it controls. To keep patients relaxed and comfortable during procedures, phlebotomists should know the basics of the neurological system.

All four bodily systems—the lungs, digestive tract, kidneys, and endocrine system—work together to keep you alive and well. Phlebotomists benefit from knowledge of these systems because it helps them anticipate how particular diseases or medications would affect a patient during a venipuncture.

When taking samples from particular patient populations, such pregnant women or people of reproductive age, it is vital to take into account the reproductive system.

Blood and the circulatory system it supports are at the heart of phlebotomy. Phlebotomists need to have a thorough familiarity with blood chemistry, the coagulation process, and the anatomy and physiology of blood arteries. This information is vital for obtaining reliable blood samples, avoiding difficulties, and spotting the warning signs of irregular clotting or bleeding disorders.

The relevance of anatomical knowledge to phlebotomy will be stressed throughout this chapter. Phlebotomists' knowledge of human anatomy helps them take accurate blood samples from patients with minimal pain and risk of contamination. Phlebotomists can better care for their patients as a whole when they have the ability to recognize anatomical differences or abnormalities that may affect venipuncture.

Phlebotomists can improve their skills, offer patients with competent and safe care, and contribute to the success of healthcare teams by learning the fundamentals of human anatomy.

Anatomical Terms

Accurately defining the position, placement, and relationship of structures within the human body requires the use of specialized words drawn from the field of anatomy. By standardizing on these phrases, medical practitioners can have more fruitful and precise conversations with one another. List of important anatomical words

Anatomical Position

The anatomical position is the default reference point for the human body. The arms are at the sides, palms facing forward, and the body is standing tall and facing forward. In this orientation, the relative positions of various body parts can be more easily described.

Anterior and Posterior

The terms "anterior" and "posterior" describe the relative positions of the front and back of the body, respectively.

Superior and Inferior

The term "superior" is used to describe a structure's location at or near the head, whereas "inferior" describes its location at or near the feet.

Proximal and Distal

A structure is said to be proximal if it is at the point of attachment or the body's center, and distal if it is far from either of those locations.

Medial and Lateral

A structure is said to be medial if it is located closer to the body's midline, and lateral if it is located further from the center.

Superficial and Deep

A superficial structure is one that is relatively close to the body's surface, whereas a deep structure is one that is significantly deeper into the body.

Dorsal and Ventral

Dorsal and ventral, respectively, relate to the rear and top of an organism or structure, and the front and bottom, respectively.

Flexion and Extension

The term "extension" is used to describe the opposite movement from "flexion," in which the angle between two bones or body components is widened.

Abduction and Adduction

A bodily part is said to be abducted when it is moved away from the body's midline and is said to be adducted when it is brought closer to the midline.

Rotation

When a body part rotates, it moves counterclockwise around its own axis.

Integumentary System

The skin, hair, nails, and related glands make up the integumentary system of the body. It prevents harmful substances from penetrating the body and protecting vital organs. The integumentary system consists of the following major components:

Skin

The skin is the body's largest organ and is composed of the outermost epidermis, the deeper dermis, and the subcutaneous tissue. It's a physical barrier that prevents things like water loss, virus entry, and harm. The skin also contains sensory receptors, helps control internal body temperature, and produces vitamin D.

Hair

Keratin makes up hair, which develops from follicles in the dermis. It can block harmful UV rays, insulate against cold, and heighten awareness, among other things.

Nails

Hard keratin is what makes up nails, which develop from the nail matrix at the nail's bed. They shield the hands from harm and improve the sensitivity of the fingertips.

Glands

Glands, such as sweat and sebaceous glands, are part of the integumentary system. The sweat glands secrete perspiration to cool the body down, while the sebaceous glands generate sebum, an oily substance that keeps the skin and hair supple and healthy.

The integumentary system is essential for homeostasis and for shielding the organism from external threats. Phlebotomists' work is greatly influenced by the integumentary system, so it's important for them to know how the skin works.

Skeletal System

The skeleton is the body's supporting structure and is made up of bones, cartilage, ligaments, and tendons. It aids in the transport of minerals and the storage of blood cells, as well as in providing support for these processes. Phlebotomists must have a strong knowledge of bone anatomy in order to properly locate veins for venipuncture. Important information regarding the skeleton is as follows:

Bones

The living tissues that form bones are stiff, yet dynamic organs. They hold the body together, shield the internal organs, and connect the muscles. The femur and humerus are examples of long bones, the carpals and tarsals are examples of short bones, the skull and the scapula are examples of flat bones, the vertebrae and the pelvis are examples of irregular bones, and the patella is an example of a sesamoid bone. There are distinct parts to every bone, such as the shaft (diaphysis), the ends (epiphysis), and the center hollow (periosteum) that houses the bone marrow.

Joints

Movement is made possible by the joints that connect bones. In terms of mobility, joints can either be fixed (synarthroses), somewhat mobile (amphiarthroses), or fully mobile (diarthroses). Hinge joints (such as the elbow), ball-and-socket joints (such as the hip), and pivot joints (such as the atlas-axis joint in the neck) are all examples of joints.

Cartilage

Cartilage is a type of connective tissue that serves as a cushion in the nose and ear, among other places. It cushions the bones and lessens the rubbing that can occur between them. Fibrocartilage is present in more stable regions, including the intervertebral discs, while hyaline cartilage protects the ends of bones in moveable joints.

Ligaments

Joint stability is provided by ligaments, which are bands of fibrous connective tissue that attach bones to each other. They prevent dislocations and injuries by limiting unnecessary motion.

Tendons

Muscles adhere to bones by means of tendons, which are tough bands of fibrous connective tissue. They connect muscles to bones, where the force they generate can be used to make motion possible.

Phlebotomists can avoid difficulties and injuries by using their knowledge of the skeletal system to locate safe venipuncture sites using bony landmarks. The antecubital fossa, on the front of the elbow, is a typical venipuncture location because many veins are situated there close to the bone.

Muscular System

The musculoskeletal system facilitates mobility, stability, heat generation, and postural maintenance. There are three distinct muscle groups that make up the body: skeletal, smooth, and cardiac. Information you need to know about the musculoskeletal system:

Skeletal Muscles

Skeletal muscles, which are connected to the bones via tendons, allow us to voluntarily move our skeletons. The agonist contracts as the antagonist relaxes, and the two muscles in a pair or group work together to accomplish this. The arrangement of muscle fibers gives skeletal muscles their distinctive striped look, known as striations.

Smooth Muscles

The linings of organs, blood arteries, and the lungs all include smooth muscles. They are in charge of involuntary actions including the narrowing of blood vessels and the tightening of the intestines.

Cardiac Muscles

The walls of the heart are made up of cardiac muscles. They are in charge of synchronized muscle contractions that circulate blood throughout the body. Involuntary regulation and properties shared with skeletal muscles characterize the cardiac muscles.

Muscle Contraction

When muscle fibers shorten and produce force, this is called a contraction. The tension between actin and myosin filaments in individual muscle cells regulates this process. Movement and the generation of the force necessary for venipuncture operations rely on this process, which is regulated by signals from the neurological system.

Muscle Groups

Movements need the coordinated efforts of many different muscle groups throughout the body. Phlebotomists must be aware of the position and movements of these muscle groups in order to choose safe venipuncture sites and keep patients comfortable. Upper-arm major muscle groups consist of the biceps and triceps, thigh major muscle groups comprise the quadriceps and hamstrings, and calf major muscle groups consist of the gastrocnemius and soleus.

Muscle Function and Posture

Muscles are not only essential for movement, but also for proper posture and stability. Together, they help keep the body stable and upright. Phlebotomists should be cognizant of the role that muscle function plays in maintaining appropriate posture during venipuncture to both reduce patient discomfort and maximize vein access.

Muscle Health and Injury Prevention

Phlebotomists that are familiar with the muscular system are better able to detect problems or injuries that may affect venipuncture. Phlebotomists who are aware of the most prevalent types of muscular injuries, such as strains and sprains, might modify their procedures or look for other venipuncture sites to prevent further injury.

Phlebotomists who want to be successful at venipuncture need have a thorough understanding of the human skeletal and muscular systems. With this information in hand, they may locate suitable venipuncture sites, anticipate any difficulties or constraints that may arise due to the patient's bone or muscular abnormalities, and keep the patient relaxed and safe throughout the procedure.

In addition, phlebotomists can better position patients for venipuncture and lower the risk of musculoskeletal strain or injury by knowing the role of muscles in maintaining posture and stability. Phlebotomists can improve their abilities and give better treatment for their patients if they learn about the skeletal and muscular systems.

Nervous System

The brain and other parts of the nervous system work together to regulate the body's activities. It takes in data, processes it, and then sends it to other parts of the body. As the neurological system affects patient comfort, reaction to operations, and overall safety, phlebotomists must have a thorough understanding of it. Here are some fundamentals concerning the brain and spinal cord:

Central Nervous System (CNS)

The brain and spinal cord make up the central nervous system. It processes information and coordinates the body's responses, acting as the control hub. Higher-level processes like thinking, remembering, and feeling occur in the brain, while the spinal cord acts as a communication hub between the brain and the rest of the body.

Peripheral Nervous System (PNS)

All nerves not found within the central nervous system make up the PNS. Additionally, the nervous system is split into the autonomic nervous system and the somatic nervous system. The autonomic nervous system regulates involuntary functions including heart rate, digestion, and respiration, while the somatic nervous system controls voluntary movements and relays sensory information.

Neurons

Neurons are specialized cells in the nervous system responsible for relaying action potentials, electrical signals. Neurons are cells that receive and transmit signals and feature a cell body, dendrites, and an axon. To know how signals are conveyed throughout the nervous system, one must have a firm grasp on the fundamental structure and function of neurons.

Neurotransmitters

Neurons are able to communicate with one another and with other cells via chemical messengers called neurotransmitters. In order to transfer a signal, they are secreted from the synaptic terminals of one neuron and then bind to receptors on the next neuron. Acylcholine, dopamine, serotonin, and norepinephrine are all examples of widely-used neurotransmitters.

Sensory and Motor Functions

Sensory data and movement are processed by the nervous system. Touch, warmth, and pain are just few of the sensations that can be perceived thanks to the sensory neurons that relay information from sensory receptors to the central nervous system. Communication between the central nervous system and the muscles and glands is made possible by motor neurons.

Reflexes

Reflexes are the body's natural, involuntary, and reflexive defense mechanisms. They entail a stimulus being detected by sensory neurons and then sent to motor neurons without going through the brain. Phlebotomists need to be familiar with reflexes in order to predict and address patient reactions during venipuncture.

Respiratory System

Exchange of gases between the body and the environment is facilitated by the respiratory system. It takes in oxygen and expels carbon dioxide, ensuring that cells have the oxygen they need to produce energy and that waste is effectively flushed out of the body. Additional information regarding the respiratory system is provided below.

Organs of the Respiratory System

The respiratory system consists mostly of the nasal cavity, pharynx, larynx, trachea, bronchi, bronchioles, and lungs. The nasal cavity and nose act as a filter, warming and humidifying the air before it enters the body. Both air and food travel through the throat. The vocal cords and the ability to make sound are housed in the larynx. The windpipe (trachea) extends from the larynx down into the lungs, where it joins the bronchi and, eventually, the even smaller bronchioles. Gas exchange takes place in the alveoli, which are tiny air sacs at the end of the bronchioles.

Gas Exchange

Alveoli serve as sites for gas exchange. When we breathe in, oxygen from the air we've just taken in diffuses across the alveolar walls and into the surrounding capillaries, where it binds to hemoglobin and is carried to every cell in our body. Carbon dioxide, a byproduct of cellular respiration, is also expelled by diffusion from the capillaries into the alveoli.

Mechanics of Breathing

The act of taking in air and releasing it again is known as breathing or ventilation. The diaphragm and intercostal muscles are the primary respiratory muscle groups responsible for its movement. Air is pulled into the lungs as the thoracic cavity is enlarged by the contraction of the diaphragm and its downward movement as the intercostal muscles expand the rib cage. The diaphragm and intercostal muscles loosen up during exhalation, allowing the lungs to recoil elastically and push air out of the body.

Respiratory Control

The brainstem's respiratory control centers, including the medulla oblongata and the pons, are responsible for regulating breathing. Chemoreceptors, which measure blood oxygen, carbon dioxide, and pH, feed information to these hubs. They regulate their breathing rate and depth to keep their gas levels stable and their blood oxygenated.

Respiratory Disorders

The respiratory system can become dysfunctional due to a variety of respiratory illnesses. Asthma, COPD, pneumonia, and other respiratory diseases and illnesses are only a few examples. Phlebotomists need to be aware of these conditions and any additional care or precautions that should be taken before, during, or after venipuncture.

Phlebotomists' knowledge of the respiratory system is critical since it affects patients' well-being during venipuncture. For normal physiological functioning and patient comfort, oxygenation is crucial. Phlebotomists need to check patients' breathing, place them in a comfortable posture to breathe easily, and watch for any signs of respiratory distress both during and after the procedure.

In addition, phlebotomists can assist their patients relax and endure venipuncture with less difficulty by instructing them in good breathing practices, such as taking calm, deep breaths. Phlebotomists can protect their patients' well-being by acknowledging the importance of the respiratory system and its function in venipuncture.

Gastrointestinal System

The gastrointestinal (GI) system, also called the digestive system, is in charge of digesting food, absorbing its nutrients, and getting rid of its byproducts. It consists of a network of organs and tissues whose coordinated efforts make digestion and absorption of food possible. Because of its potential influence on patient satisfaction and the interpretation of certain laboratory findings, phlebotomists would do well to familiarize themselves with the digestive system. Here are some fundamentals concerning the digestive tract:

Organs of the Gastrointestinal System

The digestive system consists of the oral cavity, the stomach, the proximal and distal intestines, the rectum, and the anus. Mechanical digestion begins in the mouth, where food is first chewed and then combined with saliva. After entering the stomach, it is further digested by the acid and enzymes produced there. Most nutrient absorption occurs in the small intestine, which receives food that has been partially digested from the stomach. In the large intestine, undigested food is mixed with water and electrolytes to form feces, which are then passed through the anus and rectum.

Accessory Digestive Organs

There are primary digestive organs, and then there are auxiliary organs that help in digestion. Salivary glands, liver, gallbladder, and pancreas all fall into this category. Enzymes in saliva start the digestion of carbohydrates when they are ingested. To facilitate the breakdown and absorption of fats, the liver secretes bile, which is then stored in the gallbladder before being released into the small intestine. The pancreas secretes digestive enzymes into the small intestine, where they help digest fats, proteins, and carbs even further.

Digestive Processes

Ingestion (the act of taking in food), propulsion (the action of pushing food along the digestive tract), mechanical digestion (the process of breaking down food into smaller pieces via chewing and muscular contractions), chemical digestion (the process of breaking down food into simpler molecules via enzymes and other substances), absorption (the transfer of nutrients from the digestive tract into the bloodstream), and elimination (the removal of indigestible material from the body) are all functions of the gastrointestinal system.

Roles of the Gastrointestinal System in Phlebotomy

Patient satisfaction and the interpretation of some laboratory tests may be affected by the digestive system. Some blood tests, for instance, can only provide reliable findings if the patient has fasted for a certain amount of time beforehand. Phlebotomists need to be familiar with fasting standards and provide patients with clear instructions. They should also be aware that a patient's capacity to tolerate venipuncture may be impacted by the presence of any gastrointestinal problems or symptoms.

Urinary System

The urinary system, also called the renal system, is in charge of urine's creation, storage, and excretion. It aids in maintaining proper amounts of fluids, electrolytes, and metabolic waste products excreted from the body. Phlebotomists need to know about the urinary system since it affects how they handle patients with urine disorders and how they interpret laboratory data. An overview of the urinary system is as follows:

Organs of the Urinary System

The kidneys, ureters, bladder, and urethra make up what is known as the urinary system. The kidneys are the principal organs in charge of eliminating waste from the body through urination. The ureters carry urine from the kidneys to the bladder, where it is held until it is expelled via the urethra.

Functions of the Urinary System

The urinary system is essential for eliminating waste from the body, controlling blood pressure, and maintaining fluid and electrolyte balance. The kidneys are responsible for filtering the blood and removing waste products and excess water and electrolytes while reabsorbing essential substances like glucose and electrolytes. The body's fluid and electrolyte balance is preserved by the production and evacuation of urine.

Nephrons

Kidney function is carried out by nephrons, which filter blood, reabsorb substances, and secrete waste products. Millions of nephrons, each with its own glomerulus, capillary network for filtration, and tubule system for processing filtrate, make up each kidney. The regulation of urine output by the kidneys relies on an appreciation of the anatomy and function of nephrons.

Urine Formation

Glycoprotein filtration in the kidneys, tubular reabsorption, and tubular secretion all contribute to urine production. Water, electrolytes, and tiny molecules in the blood are separated during glomerular filtration before entering the renal tubules. As the filtrate moves through the tubules, water, glucose, electrolytes, and other chemicals are reabsorbed into the bloodstream via tubular reabsorption. Substances, such as hydrogen ions and certain medicines, are actively transported from the bloodstream into the tubules during tubular secretion and then excreted in the urine.

Regulation of Water and Electrolyte Balance

The urinary system is essential for keeping the right balance of fluids and electrolytes in the body. The kidneys control blood volume, blood pressure, and intracellular substance concentration by regulating the reabsorption and excretion of water and electrolytes. These mechanisms are regulated by hormones such antidiuretic hormone (ADH) and aldosterone.

Urinary Disorders and Laboratory Tests

Interpreting laboratory tests, such as a urinalysis, often necessitates knowledge of the urinary system. Kidney function, urinary tract infections, the presence of chemicals like glucose or proteins, and other characteristics that may affect patient health can all be determined through urinalysis. Phlebotomists may need to collect urine samples for laboratory testing, and it is important for them to have a thorough understanding of the urinary system to do so safely and effectively.

Endocrine System

The endocrine system is a network of glands that release hormones into the bloodstream to control and balance body processes. It's essential for a number of processes, including maturation, metabolism, reproduction, and resistance to stress. As the endocrine system affects patient wellness, hormone levels, and the interpretation of certain laboratory tests, phlebotomists need to have a firm grasp of this physiological system. Important information regarding the endocrine system is as follows:

Glands, Endocrine

Several glands dispersed throughout the body make up what is known as the endocrine system. Pituitary, thyroid, parathyroid, adrenal, pancreatic, ovary (in females), and testes (in men) are the principal endocrine glands. Different hormones are produced by various glands to control various bodily processes.

Hormones

Endocrine glands secrete hormones into the bloodstream to act as chemical messengers. They move to their intended organs or cells, where they attach to receptors to trigger a response. Growth, metabolism, reproduction, stress response, electrolyte balance, and blood sugar management are all governed by hormones.

Hypothalamus and Pituitary Gland

The pituitary gland's hormone production is regulated by the hypothalamus in the brain. Often called the "master gland," the pituitary gland secretes hormones that regulate the activity of other endocrine glands. It's essential for proper development, metabolism, reproduction, and reaction to stress.

Thyroid and Parathyroid Glands

Hormones secreted by the thyroid gland control metabolic rate and physical development. Thyroxine (T4) and triiodothyronine (T3) are two of the hormones secreted by the thyroid gland. Calcium and phosphorus levels in the blood are controlled by parathyroid hormone (PTH), which is produced by the parathyroid glands.

Adrenal Glands

Hormones involved in stress response and electrolyte balance management are produced by the adrenal glands, which sit atop the kidneys. The adrenal cortex is responsible for the production of several important hormones, including cortisol (which aids the body's response to stress) and aldosterone (which controls the body's salt and potassium levels). The "fight or flight" reaction involves the hormones adrenaline (epinephrine) and noradrenaline (norepinephrine), both of which are produced by the adrenal medulla.

Pancreas

Both endocrine and exocrine functions are performed by the pancreas. It is an endocrine gland that controls blood sugar by secreting insulin and glucagon. Insulin reduces blood sugar levels, while glucagon raises them when necessary.

Phlebotomists need knowledge of the endocrine system since hormone levels can affect the results of some laboratory tests. Fasting requirements for certain tests may be affected by hormonal swings, therefore phlebotomists should be aware of this possibility. Patients' responses to venipuncture and general health might be affected by endocrine illnesses including diabetes and thyroid dysfunction, which your staff should be aware of.

Reproductive System

Gametes (sex cells) and the continuation of the human race are products of the reproductive system. Sexual reproductive anatomy encompasses the gonads, accessory glands, and external genitalia, among other features. Phlebotomists should have a basic knowledge of the reproductive system because it could affect patient safety, privacy, and the interpretation of certain lab findings. The fundamentals of the reproductive system are as follows:

Male Reproductive System

The testes, epididymis, vas deferens, seminal vesicles, prostate gland, and penis make up the male reproductive system. The sperm needed for fertilization is produced and transported by the male reproductive system. More information on the male reproductive system is provided below.

Testes

Spermatogenesis, the process by which sperm cells are generated, takes place primarily in the testes, the primary male reproductive organs. The male reproductive system and secondary sexual traits cannot develop in young men without the hormone testosterone, which is produced by these cells.

Epididymis

Each testis is covered by a coiled tube called the epididymis. It's where sperm go to develop into mature cells with swimming abilities and mature into storage.

Vas Deferens

Maturated sperm go from the epididymis to the ejaculatory ducts through a muscular tube called the vas deferens. The vas deferens tightens during ejaculation, directing sperm toward the urethra.

Seminal Vesicles, Prostate Gland, and Bulbourethral Glands

Fluids from these ductless glands combine with sperm to make semen. Fructose and other nutrients are provided by the seminal vesicles to the sperm. The prostate gland produces a milky fluid that buffers the pH of the vaginal canal. Before the release of semen during ejaculation, the bulbourethral glands secrete a transparent, lubricating fluid.

Penis

Men's genitalia are exposed via the penis. Shaft, glans, and the meatus of the urethra make up this structure. The penis raises when a man is sexually aroused so that sperm can enter the female reproductive system more easily.

Female Reproductive System

The ova (eggs) and the uterine environment necessary for fertilization, implantation, and embryonic development are products of the female reproductive system. More information about the female reproductive system is provided below.

Ovaries

Ovaries play a crucial role in female reproduction. Both estrogen and progesterone, the female sex hormones, are secreted by these cells. Ovulation is the process through which eggs are discharged from the ovaries.

Fallopian Tubes

Eggs that are produced during ovulation are collected by the fallopian tubes, also known as the uterine tubes. The egg needs a method to get from the ovary to the uterus, and this is what they offer. When sperm and an egg interact, fertilization usually takes place in the fallopian tubes.

Uterus

During pregnancy, a fetus grows and develops inside the uterus, often known as the womb. The uterus is a muscular organ. The uterine lining is lost during menstruation if fertilization does not take place.

Cervix

The cervix is the portion of the uterus closest to the vaginal opening. It generates mucus with varying viscosity during the menstrual cycle, which acts as a barrier when not in ovulation but lets sperm through during that period.

Vagina

The vagina is a musculoskeletal passageway that women use to give birth. During sexual interaction, it also receives the penis.

Breasts

The breasts have an important function beyond reproduction: they are a primary source of food for newborns who are breastfed. Milk-making mammary glands are found in them.

Phlebotomists should have some familiarity with the female reproductive system because of the potential effects it can have on patient safety, privacy, and the scheduling of certain diagnostic procedures. Phlebotomists need to be cognizant of the fact that a patient's health and test results may be affected by fluctuating hormone levels associated with the menstrual cycle. Patients undergoing venipuncture treatments should be provided with a safe and supportive atmosphere that respects their privacy and cultural beliefs about reproductive health.

Circulatory System

The cardiovascular system, or circulatory system, is in charge of distributing blood, nutrition, oxygen, hormones, and waste products to all parts of the body. Heart, blood arteries, and blood are its constituent parts. As phlebotomists perform venipuncture and analyze laboratory test findings, they must have a firm grasp of the circulatory system. More information about the cardiovascular system is provided below.

Heart

The heart is an organ made of muscle that can be found in the chest, slightly off-center to the left side. It functions as a pump, driving blood through the cardiovascular system. There are two atriums and two ventricles in the heart. The atria are responsible for taking in blood that is pumped back to the heart via the ventricles. The left side of the heart pumps oxygenated blood to the rest of the body, while the right side receives deoxygenated blood from the body and sends it to the lungs to be oxygenated.

Blood Vessels

Arteries, veins, and capillaries make up the body's circulatory system.

Arteries

The arterial system is responsible for transporting oxygenated blood from the heart to the rest of the body's organs and tissues. They can resist high blood pressure thanks to their thick, muscular walls and continue to pump blood even when the heart contracts. Arterioles are the tiny offshoots of arteries.

Veins

Deoxygenated blood travels through veins back to the heart from the body's tissues. They feature valves to prevent blood from flowing backwards and thinner walls than arteries. Veins are the blood vessels responsible for transporting blood back to the heart.

Capillaries

Connecting arterioles and venules are microscopic, thin-walled blood arteries called capillaries. They allow for communication between the circulatory system and the rest of the body. Diffusion of oxygen, nutrients, and waste items from the blood to the cells is made possible by capillaries.

Blood

The blood that flows through our veins and arteries is a specialized connective tissue. It has multiple parts, including the following:

Plasma

About 55% of the total volume of blood is plasma, the liquid component of blood. Water, proteins, hormones, nutrients, waste materials, and other components make up this yellowish fluid. Plasma is essential for carrying these chemicals to their respective locations in the body.

Red Blood Cells (RBCs)

The erythrocyte, or red blood cell, is the most common type of blood cell. Their principal role is to carry oxygen from the lungs to the rest of the body and carbon dioxide from the tissues back to the lungs to be exhaled. Hemoglobin, found in RBCs, is the oxygen-binding protein responsible for blood's characteristic red color.

White Blood Cells (WBCs)

Leukocytes, or white blood cells, are an important part of the immune system's ability to fight off illnesses and infections. They are useful for detecting and eliminating unwanted microorganisms, chemicals, and cells.

Platelets

Platelets, also known as thrombocytes, are fragments of larger cells that help the blood to clot and stop bleeding. They clump together at the site of an injury and seal it up by adhering to blood arteries that have been damaged.

Phlebotomists rely heavily on venipuncture, which is intimately related to the circulatory system.

The Coagulation Process

Clotting of blood, or hemostasis, is a complex mechanism that stops bleeding when a blood artery is damaged. A stable blood clot forms after a sequence of stages and the activation of several chemicals. The coagulation process is described in greater depth below.

Vasoconstriction

Vasoconstriction, or the narrowing of the blood vessel walls, occurs when a blood vessel is injured. By restricting blood flow to the damaged location, this helps keep blood loss to a minimum.

Formation of Platelet Plug

When a blood vessel is damaged, platelets are among the first responders. They congregate at the site of vessel injury and stick together to create a plug called a platelet plug. The clotting process is aided by the chemical signals and chemicals released by platelets.

Coagulation Cascade

Fibrin, the primary component of blood clots, is formed through a sequence of enzyme events known as the coagulation cascade. It's segmented into the intrinsic and extrinsic routes, both of which eventually merge into one.

Intrinsic Pathway

When collagen is exposed because vessel walls have been broken, the intrinsic route is set in motion. Factor X is activated as a result of this exposure, which sets off a chain reaction involving other clotting factors.

Extrinsic Pathway

Tissue factor (TF) is a chemical secreted by injured tissues that triggers the extrinsic route. Activation of factor X requires the formation of a complex between TF and factor VII.

Common Pathway

Prothrombinase is an enzyme formed when factor X is combined with factor V, calcium ions, and platelet phospholipids. The enzyme prothrombinase catalyzes the conversion of prothrombin to thrombin. Fibrin is formed when the soluble protein fibrinogen is cleaved by the coagulation factor thrombin. When fibrin strands combine, a mesh-like structure is created that can ensnare and hold various blood components such as platelets, RBCs, and more. By forming a clot, this mesh stops bleeding and sets the stage for the wound to heal.

Clot Retraction and Serum Formation

When the platelets in a clot begin to contract after it has formed, the clot becomes smaller and more compact. Clot retraction describes this phenomenon. Serum, a transparent, protein-rich fluid, is forced out as the clot contracts. Different proteins and growth factors found in serum speed up the recovery process.

Fibrinolysis

The fibrinolysis mechanism begins to disintegrate the clot once the injured blood vessel has been healed. Fibrin is degraded into smaller fragments known as fibrin degradation products by the enzyme plasmin. This makes it possible for blood flow to be gradually restored and the clot components to be gradually removed.

In order to prevent either excessive clotting or bleeding, the coagulation process is strictly controlled. The balance between clot formation and clot dissolution is controlled by multiple variables, including platelets, clotting factors, and regulatory proteins. Disorders of blood clotting and excessive bleeding can result from an imbalance here.

Blood Vessels

In order to transfer blood and allow for the exchange of oxygen, nutrients, waste products, and hormones with tissues and organs, a network of tubular structures called blood vessels is present throughout the body. Arteries, veins, and capillaries are the three major branches of the circulatory system. As they work directly with blood arteries during venipuncture, phlebotomists must have a thorough knowledge of their anatomy and physiology. Here are some other facts regarding blood vessels:

Arteries

Arteries are large blood veins with strong walls that transport oxygenated blood from the heart to the body's tissues and organs. They are able to resist high blood pressure thanks to the elastic fibers and smooth muscle in their walls. Arterioles are tiny branches of arteries that carry blood to more specific areas.

Veins

Veins are the blood arteries responsible for returning oxygen-poor blood from the tissues back to the heart. They feature valves to prevent blood from flowing backwards and thinner walls than arteries. The smooth muscle and elasticity of veins are both lower than those of arteries. Veins begin as a network of smaller blood vessels called venules.

Capillaries

Connecting arterioles and venules, capillaries are the tiniest and most delicate blood vessels. They connect blood vessels throughout tissues, facilitating the transport of oxygen, nutrients, and waste materials. Substances diffuse more easily through capillary walls because they are made up of a single layer of endothelial cells.

Microcirculation

Exchange of chemicals between the blood and tissues, also known as microcirculation, takes place at the capillary level. Transporting oxygen and nutrients to cells and eliminating waste materials are two of its most important functions. Diffusion across the capillary walls facilitates the exchange.

Vascular System Regulation

The autonomic nervous system, hormones, and local factors such chemical signals secreted by tissues all play a role in controlling blood vessel diameter. When blood arteries constrict, blood flow decreases, and when they dilate, blood flow increases. This control allows the body to maintain a steady blood pressure, target blood flow to specific areas, and adapt to changing conditions.

Phlebotomists must have an intimate familiarity with the anatomy and physiology of blood vessels in order to perform a successful venipuncture. They have to think about the patient's convenience and ease of access while deciding where to draw blood. Phlebotomists who are well-versed in vascular anatomy are better able to spot dangers, such as the risk of arterial puncture, and prevent them.

Coagulation and Hemostasis

Coagulation and hemostasis are complex processes that aid one another in stopping bleeding and forming clots. Proteins, platelets, and clotting factors all work together to bring about these events. As they work directly with blood during venipuncture, phlebotomists must have a thorough understanding of the processes involved in coagulation and hemostasis. Here is a comprehensive breakdown of the processes of coagulation and hemostasis:

Platelet Activation and Formation of the Platelet Plug

Platelets are activated and migrate to the site of a blood vessel injury. The release of von Willebrand factor (vWF) and exposure of the subendothelial connective tissue set off this process. Next, the platelets undergo a morphological transformation, spreading out filopodia and pseudopodia to form clusters. Adenosine diphosphate (ADP), thromboxane A2 (TXA2), and serotonin are some of the chemicals released by activated platelets that serve to recruit additional platelets to the area of injury. In doing so, a platelet plug is formed, which aids in temporarily sealing the broken blood channel.

Coagulation Cascade

Clotting factors undergo a sequence of enzymatic processes known as the coagulation cascade, which ultimately results in the creation of fibrin. It has three distinct branches: the intrinsic, the extrinsic, and the common.

Intrinsic Pathway

When blood contacts an injured surface, such collagen exposed at the site of vascular injury, the intrinsic pathway is set in motion. Factor XII (Hageman factor) is activated by this stimulus, and further processes involving factors XI, IX, and VIII begin.

Extrinsic Pathway

Tissue factor, also known as factor III, is released from non-vascular injured tissue, setting off a chain of events known as the extrinsic route. Factor X (Stuart-Prower factor) is activated when TF combines with factor VII (proconvertin) to create a complex.

Common Pathway

In order to create prothrombinase, factor X must first be activated, at which point it combines with factor V (proaccelerin), calcium ions, and platelet phospholipids. Thrombin (factor IIa) is the active form of the protein prothrombin (factor II), which is converted to by prothrombinase. The soluble protein fibrinogen is cleaved by the coagulation agent thrombin to form fibrin. The platelet plug is stabilized and a clot is formed when fibrin strands polymerize and cross-link to form a three-dimensional meshwork.

Clot Retraction and Serum Formation

When a blood clot forms, the platelets within it contract to make the clot smaller and denser. Clot retraction describes this phenomenon. Serum, a transparent fluid rich in proteins, is expelled as the clot contracts. Different proteins and growth factors found in serum speed up the recovery process.

Fibrinolysis

The fibrinolysis mechanism begins to disintegrate the blood clot after the injured blood vessel has been healed. Fibrin is degraded into smaller fragments known as fibrin degradation products by the enzyme plasmin. To produce plasmin, plasminogen must be converted into its active form by tissue plasminogen activator (tPA). Blood flow can be gradually restored by fibrinolysis, and the clot components can be removed.

Excessive clotting or bleeding can be prevented by the strict regulation of the coagulation and hemostasis processes. This fine equilibrium is maintained by a complex network of clotting factors, regulatory proteins, and inhibitors.

Chapter 5

Patient Preparation

Patient preparation is essential in the fields of healthcare and medical diagnostics since it increases the likelihood of effective outcomes. Preparing a patient for venipuncture, the act of collecting blood from a patient for laboratory testing, is the emphasis of this chapter. Error prevention, patient safety, and accurate test findings all hinge on how well patients are prepared for their examinations.

The significance of correct patient identification is stressed at the outset of the chapter. This is a necessary precaution to ensure that specimens are collected and analyzed correctly. Proper patient identification is stressed, such as by verifying the patient's wristband or confirming the patient's identity verbally.

Patient preparation also includes filling out the necessary requisition paperwork. These forms assist make sure the right tests are done by providing essential information regarding the tests ordered by the healthcare provider. This chapter outlines why it's crucial to provide accurate information while filling out a request form, as well as the consequences for doing otherwise during the testing procedure.

Involuntary venipuncture is a medical treatment that requires informed consent from the patient. The importance of getting the patient's or their legal guardian's permission to do a venipuncture is stressed in this chapter. Explaining the procedure, dangers, and benefits to the patient is stressed as a means of gaining their trust and cooperation during the process.

The materials needed for venipuncture, or blood collection, are then covered in detail. Needles, collecting tubes, antibiotics, tourniquets, and gloves are all examples of such supplies. Patient safety and the avoidance of cross-contamination are prioritized throughout this chapter, which highlights the significance of utilizing sterile and appropriate equipment.

Choosing the correct venipuncture site is essential. Identifying a suitable vein for blood collection is a crucial step. Access to veins, patient comfort, and the possibility of complications are all discussed in this chapter as they pertain to making the all-important site choice. In addition, it includes instructions for how to clean the incision site thoroughly to prevent infections and hematomas.

Detailed instructions on how to perform a venipuncture are provided in this chapter. It discusses how the patient should be positioned, how the needle should be inserted, how the blood flow should be managed, and how the tubes should be labeled. Explicit directions are given to reduce patient stress and the risk of injury during blood collection.

Instructions for filling out requisition forms are provided to stress the need of remembering to include all relevant details. This comprises the patient's name, address, date of birth, insurance information, healthcare provider information, and test requests. This chapter focuses on the importance of requisition forms in ensuring accurate test identification, timely reporting of results, and clear lines of communication between medical staff.

Successful venipuncture relies heavily on the patient's posture. This chapter instructs healthcare providers on how to best posture patients for blood draws while they are seated, lying down, or standing. Patient comfort, venous access, and procedure efficiency can all be improved with the right placement.

There are a number of factors that can affect how blood samples are taken. Patient age, medical history, medications, hydration levels, and circadian rhythms are just some of the topics covered in this chapter. To properly interpret laboratory test findings and provide optimal patient care, an appreciation of these factors is crucial.

The context of venipuncture is also examined in terms of special considerations. Considerations such as patient allergies, potential consequences (such as vasovagal responses), and age-related needs are important in this context. Patient safety and quality specimens can both be maximized if these guidelines are followed.

Testing requirements are briefly discussed in this chapter, with an emphasis on the necessity of strictly adhering to all given protocols in the laboratory. Instructions for obtaining valid and trustworthy test findings are emphasized, with particular attention paid to fasting requirements, specimen collection timing, and sample processing.

This chapter also discusses the collecting of non-blood specimens. While venipuncture is the major method discussed in this chapter, other specimen types such as urine, saliva, and tissue samples are also acknowledged. It stresses the significance of using correct collection methods and labeling and treatment of specimens.

The need of collecting a sufficient sample for testing is emphasized by discussing minimum and maximum collection amounts. The guidelines in this chapter will help you collect the appropriate amount of blood or other specimens for your test.

The chapter finishes with a discussion of important takeaways for preparing patients for venipuncture. It reviews the chapter's discussion of the crucial procedures, factors, and conditions that must be met to guarantee a successful blood collection, reliable test results, and patient safety.

Healthcare providers can improve the venipuncture process, the patient's experience, and the delivery system as a whole by adhering to established protocols and guidelines for patient preparation.

Identifying the Patient

Patient safety, error prevention, and proper care all depend on correct identification, making it a top priority in healthcare settings. There are several options for checking a patient's identity.

Checking the patient's wristband is a regular practice. In addition to the patient's entire name and birth date, this band may also include a special identifier. The information on the wristband should be double-checked with the patient's verbal affirmation to guarantee correctness.

The patient's entire name and birth date can also be a useful piece of information. This acts as an oral confirmation and can be checked against the patient's official records or other forms of identification.

A two-person verification approach may be used in emergency situations or during high-risk processes. To reduce the possibility of patient misidentification, this procedure requires two healthcare providers to independently verify the patient's identity.

It is also crucial to have open lines of contact with the patient. Patients are more likely to cooperate with the verification procedure if they are addressed by name and informed of its aim. If a patient has any questions or concerns about their identification or the upcoming operation, healthcare providers should urge them to speak up.

Requisition Forms

Laboratory personnel rely heavily on requisition forms to ensure they are conducting the correct tests as requested by the healthcare provider. The relevant tests will be run and reliable findings will be acquired if requisition forms are filled out correctly and completely.

It's crucial to include all relevant patient details when filling out request papers. The complete name of the patient, the patient's date of birth, the patient's gender, and any pertinent medical history that may affect test interpretation are all examples of this. Delays, mistakes, or further tests may need to be performed because of inaccurate or insufficient data.

Specific test codes or names are an essential part of request forms. A specific name or code is given to each laboratory test to ensure correct identification. Providers of medical services should double-check that the requisition form has the proper test codes or names. This aids in avoiding misunderstandings and guarantees accurate testing.

Requisition forms should include all pertinent patient and test data, as well as any pertinent special instructions or prerequisites. If fasting is needed before a certain test, for instance, that needs to be specified on the form. Similarly, the requisition form should make it crystal apparent if there are any special instructions for collecting, handling, or transporting the samples. This aids laboratory workers in following proper procedures and guarantees reliable testing.

Consent

Informed consent is a cornerstone of both medical ethics and the law. Patients are given the tools they need to make educated decisions about their treatment, including invasive procedures like venipuncture.

Healthcare providers should use plain language while explaining the venipuncture method to patients in order to gain their trust and cooperation. They need to talk about why the procedure is being done, what might go wrong, what might go right, and what other choices they have. By giving them this knowledge, patients may decide for themselves whether or not to go through with the treatment.

The patient's level of comprehension of the material presented must be determined. Medical staff should encourage patients to voice any concerns they may have by asking questions. This aids in making sure that patients fully understand the surgery, its potential outcomes, and any risks involved.

If the patient lacks the requisite mental or physical faculties to give consent, a legal guardian or other legally appointed representative may do so on their behalf. A parent or legal guardian, for example, should have full decision-making authority for their child. Healthcare providers are obligated to confirm the representative's authority and record their findings.

Consent documentation is an important part of the consent procedure. The technique should be discussed, the patient's understanding should be evaluated, and consent should be sought before the procedure is documented in the patient's medical record. Patients may be required to sign a consent form as an extra layer of documentation in some circumstances.

Consent is not a one-and-done kind of thing. Patients are free to revoke their permission at any moment. The withdrawal of permission should be documented in the patient's medical record and the choice should be respected and honored by healthcare providers.

In conclusion, preparing a patient for venipuncture requires correct patient identification, complete requisition documents, and get informed consent. These measures help keep patients safe, guarantee accurate testing, and adhere to all applicable laws and regulations in the healthcare industry.

Venipuncture Equipment

Safe and effective blood collection requires the use of appropriate venipuncture equipment. The essential tools for performing a venipuncture are as follows:

Venipuncture is only possible with specialized needles made for drawing blood. Needles come in a wide range of sizes, most commonly denoted by the gauge number. Needle sizes are described by their gauge, with smaller numbers indicating thinner needles. Needles with gauges of 20, 21, and 22 are frequently used for venipuncture. Needles with a bigger gauge are used on patients with larger or more accessible veins, while thinner needles are reserved for those with more delicate or smaller veins. Depending on the size and health of the patient's veins, the right needle size must be chosen.

Blood samples are collected and stored in collection tubes. varied types of testing require varied sizes and chemical compositions of these tubes. Anticoagulant- or clot-activator-containing collection tubes are frequently used. Examples include EDTA, citrate, and heparin. The healthcare provider's test orders will dictate which collecting tube is used.

A tourniquet is a device used to temporarily stop blood flow to a vein so that a venipuncture can be performed. Proximal to the chosen venipuncture site, a large elastic band or blood pressure cuff is wrapped around the patient's upper arm. The tourniquet is used to expand the veins so that needles can be easily inserted into them. However, after finding a good vein and before inserting the needle, you should quickly relax the tourniquet to prevent venous stasis and possible specimen contamination.

To reduce the likelihood of an infection spreading, antiseptics are used to clean the venipuncture site prior to needle insertion. Alcohol, chlorhexidine, and iodine-based solutions are all commonly used as antiseptics. Before inserting the needle, follow the manufacturer's recommendations for applying the chosen antiseptic and wait for it to dry completely.

Aseptic procedure and the avoidance of cross-contamination necessitate the use of disposable gloves during venipuncture. By separating the healthcare provider's hands from the patient's blood, gloves help prevent the spread of infection. Gloves should be the right size to allow for a good fit and maximum dexterity during the process.

Needle and syringe sharps should be disposed of in a puncture-resistant, leak-proof sharps container. After a venipuncture is complete, the needle should be disposed of in a sharps container to reduce the risk of needlestick accidents and keep the workplace secure.

Site Selection

The success of blood collection and the patient's level of discomfort can both be affected by where the venipuncture is performed. The age, health, vein accessibility, and reason for the blood sample all play a role in determining the best venipuncture site. Venipuncture is typically performed at:

The antecubital fossa, found at the inside of the elbow, is the most popular venipuncture site. It has several veins, including the cephalic vein, basilic vein, and median cubital vein. The median cubital vein, which may be found in the middle of the antecubital fossa, is a popular choice because of its visibility and reliability.

When the antecubital fossa veins are unusable or damaged, the dorsal hand veins may be used as an alternative. Veins on the back of the hand are often easy to see and reach, making them a good choice for venipuncture. However, the patient may have more pain or discomfort at this location.

In addition to the cephalic vein and basilic vein, the veins in the forearm can be used for venipuncture. These veins tend to be more noticeable in those who have strengthened their muscles significantly or in specific patient populations.

In some cases, when other sites are not an option, such as when giving blood, the patient's wrist or ankle veins can be used instead. Since these veins are smaller and more prone to difficulties, venipuncture at them must be carefully planned.

Site preference is affected by the patient's age and medical history. The dorsal foot veins and the scalp veins are also viable options for pediatric patients. Veins in the hand or forearm are commonly used because they are easily accessible and rather stable, even in older or frail individuals.

Healthcare providers should evaluate the veins' size, depth, and tortuosity in addition to their overall health and visibility before deciding where to do a venipuncture. Venipuncture is most successful with veins that are firm, palpable, and resilient.

How to Perform Venipuncture

To guarantee patient satisfaction, precise blood collection, and compliance with all relevant safety measures, venipuncture must be performed in a methodical fashion. The standard stages for doing a venipuncture are as follows:

1. **The doctor must first:** Confirm the patient's identify by introducing yourself. Describe the process and answer their questions. Lie the patient down or have them sit in a chair with their arm outstretched and supported.

2. **Equip yourself with what you'll need:** Gather the needles, tubes for collecting blood,

tourniquet, disinfectant, gloves, and sharps container needed to perform a venipuncture. Verify that the specimen collection tubes correspond to the tests requested.

3. Maintaining good hand hygiene entails routine hand washing with soap and water or the use of an alcohol-based hand sanitizer.

4. Select a good vein, then place the tourniquet about 3 to 4 inches above where you want to do the venipuncture. The tourniquet needs to be snug enough to restrict venous blood flow but not so tight that the patient experiences pain or venous stasis.

5. **Find the vein:** Palpate the skin near the skin's surface until you find the vein you'll be using for venipuncture. Check for veins that can be seen, felt, and are relatively strong. If the veins are not easily visible, tap the region gently or warm it up.

6. Prepare the venipuncture site by scrubbing it with an antiseptic solution in a circular motion, working from the center outward. Do not touch anything until the antiseptic has dried.

7. **Get the tools ready:** Discard the packaging from the sterile needle and insert it into the collection tube. To prevent any possible contamination or mishmash of samples, fill the collecting tubes in the sequence given.

8. Hold the needle firmly and at an angle of 15 to 30 degrees with respect to the skin. Make sure the point of the needle is pointing up.

9. The needle should be inserted into the vein in a quick, even motion. Keep your needle under control and steer clear of any unnecessary probing or repositioning to prevent tissue damage.

10. Release the tourniquet as soon as blood begins to enter the collection tube to verify successful venous access. If blood is flowing steadily into the collection tube, venous access has been established.

11. Gather the necessary quantity of blood and transfer it to the designated collection tubes. If there are any instructions regarding the order of collecting, be sure to stick to them.

12. After blood has been drawn, the needle should be carefully and slowly removed from the vein. Hemostasis is achieved by applying mild pressure with sterile gauze or cotton to the venipuncture site.

13. Put the sample in a safe place and throw away the needle. Put the needle in the sharps container for disposal. Clearly identify the patient's collected tubes by labeling them with their information. To stop bleeding from the venipuncture site, apply pressure and a dressing.

14. Give the sufferer some relief by doing things like changing their bandage and keeping an eye on them. Always be on the lookout for indicators of problems, such as a hematoma forming or excessive bleeding, in the patient.

15. **Take notes about the process:** Carefully record all aspects of the venipuncture operation, from the site chosen to the tools employed, any issues experienced, and the patient's reaction.

16. The success of venipuncture, patient safety, and the quality of the sample can all be guaranteed if medical practitioners stick to these rules.

Requisition Forms Requirements

It is impossible to accurately and efficiently process laboratory tests without requisition forms. In order to ensure appropriate sample collection and result interpretation, healthcare professionals must verify that requisition forms meet certain requirements. Key items needed for a requisition form are listed below.

Complete and accurate patient information, such as full name, DOB, gender, and ID number (if relevant), must be included on all requisition forms. The relevant patient's samples can then be identified and matched with them thanks to this data.

Healthcare providers should be specific about which tests they need on the requisition form. To guarantee that the right tests are carried out, they must be clearly labeled with the appropriate test code or name.

Providing pertinent clinical information on the requisition form is essential. Clinical indications for the desired tests, existing medications, and the patient's medical history may all be included here. The laboratory personnel can better interpret the results of the ordered tests with this background information.

The sample collection date and time must be noted on the requisition form. Specific testing requirements, such as time-sensitive tests or monitoring tests, necessitate this data for tracking the timeliness of sample collection, assuring accurate result interpretation, and meeting testing standards.

Name, contact information, and signature of the ordering healthcare professional should be legible and included on the request form. In circumstances where a healthcare provider needs clarification or more information about a laboratory test result, this data facilitates efficient communication between the laboratory and the provider.

The requisition form should include explicit details on any particular instructions or considerations for sample collection, handling, or transportation. Fasting guidelines, sample collection protocols, and transportation considerations are all examples. Adherence to these guidelines guarantees that the gathered samples are accurate and complete.

All information on requisition forms must be typed or printed clearly. Test orders might be delayed, messed up, or misunderstood if forms are illegible or missing information. Providers of medical services should take extra precaution to fill out requisition forms accurately and include all pertinent data.

Patient Positioning

Venipuncture success and patient comfort depend on the patient being positioned correctly. The patient's arm or hand position plays a significant role in how easily the veins may be seen and accessed. Important factors to keep in mind when placing a patient for a venipuncture are as follows:

Patients can be positioned seated or lying down, depending on the patient's preference and the preference of the healthcare professional. Routine venipuncture is typically performed while the patient is seated because it allows them to remain in a comfortable, relaxed position and provides convenient access to the antecubital fossa. However, for the sake of patient safety, lying down may be preferable in some cases, such as with patients who are prone to vasovagal syncope.

Whether on a flat surface, a pillow, or an armrest, the patient's arm should be extended and supported. This makes it simpler to detect and access the veins by reducing muscle tension and expanding them.

The palm of the patient's hand should be facing up when deciding which hand to use as a venipuncture site. The dorsal hand veins are more readily visible and accessible. Depending on the patient's preference and the ease with which veins may be accessed, the fingers may be slightly stretched or relaxed.

The patient's elbow should be bent at a comfortable angle if the antecubital fossa is to be used as the venipuncture site. This placement stabilizes the arm and exposes the veins at the elbow bend for easier access and examination.

Extra padding or support under the patient's arm or hand may be necessary to ensure a relaxed and comfortable position for venipuncture in some people. Patients with limited mobility or problems affecting joint stability may benefit from the added cushioning and support provided by a pillow or folded towel.

Patient posture should focus on maximizing vein visibility and access without compromising patient comfort or compliance. If the patient has any physical restrictions or special needs, the healthcare professional should discuss these factors with the patient to establish the best position for venipuncture.

Variables Impacting Collection

The procedure and outcome of drawing blood can be affected by a number of variables. If you want trustworthy test results, you need to take these into account and fix them. Some important factors that can affect sample size are as follows:

The health of the veins and the ease with which blood can be drawn are crucial factors in the success of any blood collection. Individual differences exist in vein size, depth, resilience, and visibility. Factors such as hydration status, medical problems, and venipuncture history can all have an impact on the condition of a patient's veins. Vein accessibility and condition should be taken into account when deciding where on the patient's body to do the venipuncture.

Blood collection can be affected by a number of factors relating to the patient. The fragility and availability of veins can, for example, decline with age. Veins in children may be smaller and more fragile, necessitating the use of specific methods and equipment. Venipuncture might be difficult in elderly people because of vein fragility, diminished flexibility, and reduced blood flow. Vein visibility and accessibility may also be impacted by patient variables such as obesity, edema, or scarring, necessitating alternate venipuncture techniques.

In order to avoid further bleeding and hematoma formation, it is essential to achieve hemostasis after venipuncture. It is crucial to apply sufficient pressure to the venipuncture site and ensure the formation of a durable clot. The ability of the patient to produce clots, the presence of drugs that impact coagulation, and the presence of bleeding disorders are all factors that should be taken into account when managing hemostasis.

Phlebotomy Method:

Venipuncture method makes a big difference in blood collection success. The quality and quantity of a sample may be affected by factors such as the needle's entry angle, depth, and direction, and the rate of blood flow. In order to reduce the impact of phlebotomist-introduced variations, medical professionals should stick to standard phlebotomy procedures and protocols.

Draw Order:

The order in which blood is drawn into tubes is important for maintaining sample quality and avoiding contamination. When collecting numerous tubes, it is crucial to do so in the correct order to guarantee reliable findings. The rules of the laboratory and the tests being conducted will determine the draw order.

Some substances found in the patient's body or the surrounding environment can skew the findings of laboratory tests. Alcohol and disinfectants used at the venipuncture site are two examples of pollutants that can invalidate a test. Results may also be affected by drugs, intravenous fluids, or compounds related to the patient's underlying medical condition that are present in the patient's blood. Reliable results require that as few contaminants as possible be present during sample collection.

Healthcare professionals can streamline the collection procedure, increase sample quality, and guarantee accurate test results by knowing and addressing these aspects. Taking into account patient-specifics, according to established procedures, and maintaining open lines of communication with the lab will help reduce the likelihood of error and ensure the quality of the samples you send them.

Special Considerations

Special circumstances may emerge during venipuncture and specimen collection that call for extra caution and attention. Patient populations, medical problems, and other factors that may affect the collection process are all things to think about. Specifically, you should bear in mind the following:

Venipuncture in pediatric patients calls for adapted procedures and extra care. Veins in children are typically more difficult to access because they are smaller and more brittle. To reduce patient trauma and potential consequences, medical professionals should use appropriately sized needles and procedures such the butterfly approach or syringe draw. Anxiety can be reduced and a successful collection achieved through the use of distraction strategies, parental or guardian participation, and the establishment of a child-friendly setting.

Elderly Patients:

Venipuncture can be more challenging because of the patient's age-related fragility of veins, diminished skin elasticity, and decreased blood flow. When performing a venipuncture, medical professionals should exercise caution and think about alternatives such using a smaller-gauge needle or a syringe draw. Patient comfort and safety from unnecessary bruising and bleeding can be maximized by open communication and careful management.

Patients with Difficult Veins:

Obesity, scar tissue, or a history of intravenous drug use are all potential causes of vein difficulty. In such circumstances, it may be required to use an alternative venipuncture site or method. To improve vein visibility and selection, you can move to a different area or utilize techniques like transillumination, warm compresses, or specialized vein-locating gadgets.

Some people get nervous or scared when they have to get a vein pricked. It is essential for medical professionals to reassure patients, explain the procedure in detail, and encourage open dialogue. Patients are more likely to cooperate with the collection process if they feel safe and secure in the space they are in.

It may be difficult to acquire informed permission or give clear instructions during venipuncture from individuals who are not fluent in English or who have hearing issues. Professional interpreters, translation services, and other visual aids can help healthcare providers better communicate with their patients.

Testing Requirements

Preserving specimen integrity and ensuring reliable findings from laboratory testing necessitates adhering to distinct protocols for collecting, handling, and transporting samples. The nature of the test being conducted may dictate specific needs. Some typical criteria for testing are as follows:

Some lab procedures, like lipid profiles and glucose levels, need patients to fast before collecting their samples. In order to get reliable test results, patients may be asked to fast for a certain amount of time, usually between 8 and 12 hours. Patients must be given explicit information on how long they must go without eating before to their scheduled procedure.

Time-Sensitive Tests:

Due to the stability or biological changes of the analytes being evaluated, certain tests necessitate quick sample collection and processing. Sample collection windows may be required, for instance, for tests involving volatile chemicals or hormones with diurnal fluctuations. In order to get accurate results, it's important to stick to the specified time frames.

In terms of sample volume, the minimum and maximum amounts needed for analysis will vary depending on the type of test being performed. It is the responsibility of the healthcare provider to gather enough specimen to run the necessary tests. When there isn't enough data to go around, it may be necessary to go back and get more samples.

Different types of sample collection containers or additives may be needed to maintain sample integrity for certain assays. Anticoagulant or preservative-treated tubes, for instance, may be necessary for several diagnostic procedures. In order to get reliable test findings, medical professionals should know what kind of collection containers and chemicals to use for each type of examination.

Non-Blood Specimen Collection

Diagnostic testing doesn't have to rely just on blood samples, though. Certain illnesses can be better diagnosed, monitored, and treated with the use of information gleaned from these non-blood specimens. Some alternatives to blood collection include:

Urine:

Specimens of urine are routinely taken for urinalysis, drug testing, and the diagnosis of UTIs.

Urine samples can be obtained via clean-catch midstream collection or catheterization, both of which must adhere to strict hygiene requirements to avoid contamination.

Collecting a stool sample can help diagnose a number of gastrointestinal issues such parasites, infections, and internal bleeding. Using a sterile container or a collection kit, patients may be asked to collect a tiny amount of their faeces for testing.

Saliva:

Specimens of saliva can be used for checking hormone levels, analyzing DNA, or detecting certain infections. Patients may be requested to spit into a sterile container or use saliva collection devices to deliver a sample of their saliva.

Diagnostics of respiratory illnesses including tuberculosis and pneumonia require sputum samples. Patients are prompted to cough vigorously and deposit their expectorated sputum in a clean container.

Cerebrospinal fluid (CSF):

Cerebrospinal fluid (CSF) specimens are taken during a lumbar puncture procedure to assess central nervous system diseases like meningitis and multiple sclerosis. Only qualified medical professionals should attempt this treatment due to the complexity involved.

Specimens for testing for sexually transmitted infections (STIs) are often collected using genital swabbing. The urethra, cervix, vagina, or rectum may be swabbed with a collection device and procedure particular to the test at hand.

Accurate results from the collection of non-blood specimens necessitate the use of correct methodology and adherence to established protocols. Providers of medical care should adhere to standard procedures and inform patients on proper specimen collection, including any prerequisite steps or storage needs.

Minimum and Maximum Collection Amounts

It is crucial to gather enough of a sample when sending samples to the lab so that all necessary tests may be run. There may be minimum and maximum collecting requirements that must be met for different types of specimens. Here are some things to think about when deciding how many of each sort of specimen to collect:

When collecting blood, the volume needed for the tests is usually the bare minimum that must be collected. It is crucial to collect enough blood to do all of the relevant tests, which may have varying volume needs. It is common practice to collect only as much blood as the collection tube will hold. If the maximum volume is exceeded, the ratio of blood to additive may be incorrect, which could invalidate the test.

The volume of urine needed for a certain test or analysis is usually used as the bare minimum for a collection. In order to test the analytes of interest precisely, a sufficient volume of urine must be collected. Urine collection volumes are often limited by the size of the available container and the needs of the testing facility. If the maximum volume is exceeded, the analytes may be diluted, and the results of the test may be inaccurate.

Stool:

The volume required for the proposed tests is usually the minimal collection amount for stool specimens. If only a small sample of stool is collected, there may not be enough for a thorough study. In most cases, the maximum amount of stool that may be collected is limited by the container's capacity and other logistical constraints. If the specimen's volume is too large, it may be difficult to process.

Saliva, sputum, and vaginal swabs are all examples of non-blood specimens that may have different minimum and maximum collection volumes. These specifications are often set by the laboratory's norms and the nature of the test or analysis being conducted. Adequate sample collection relies on careful adherence to the procedures outlined for each kind of material.

Key Takeaways of Patient Preparation

In order to get reliable test findings, it is essential to collect specimens from well-prepared patients. Important points to remember when preparing a patient for laboratory testing are as follows:

Accurate patient identification is crucial for avoiding duplicate samples and correctly attributing test results to the right patients. Accurate patient identification is facilitated by the use of unique identifiers including full name, date of birth, and identification numbers.

Collecting and analyzing samples correctly relies on requisition forms that have been filled out thoroughly and accurately. Patient information, test requests, clinical data, collection date and time, healthcare provider data, and any further instructions should all be included on requisition forms. The testing procedure might be streamlined with the use of legible and comprehensive requisition forms.

Obtaining patients' informed consent before to collecting specimens is crucial for upholding legal and ethical standards and respecting patients' rights. In order for patients to make educated decisions regarding their healthcare, doctors must outline the tests' goals, potential side effects, potential benefits, and alternative treatments.

Needles, syringes, and collection tubes used in venipuncture must be properly selected and sterilized to ensure a successful blood draw. Sample integrity can be protected and difficulties avoided with the right tools.

Vein accessibility and patient comfort are both improved by a properly positioned patient during venipuncture. The veins in the patient's arm or hand should be easily accessible, and the patient's muscles should be relaxed.

Collection Factors Several factors, including vein health and accessibility, patient characteristics, hemostasis, phlebotomy technique, drawing order, and interfering chemicals, might affect the quality of a given sample. Medical professionals need to think about these factors and use suitable methods to reduce their impact on sample quality.

Patients with problematic veins or communication challenges may require additional care, as may patients of all ages who are particularly frail or young. Successful specimen collection relies on adjusting collection methods to the specific needs of each patient.

Different tests have different requirements, such as fasting, time-sensitive collection, sample volume, and collecting containers. Results from tests are more likely to be accurate and trustworthy if these guidelines are followed.

Collection of Non-Blood Specimens: Many different types of non-blood specimens can be obtained for diagnostic testing in addition to blood. Accurate results can only be achieved by following established protocols when collecting non-blood specimens such urine, faeces, saliva, sputum, or genital swabs.

The quality and reliability of laboratory tests can be improved by following correct patient preparation practices, which in turn improves patient care and treatment outcomes.

Chapter 6

Routine Blood Collection

The routine collection of blood is an essential medical process that takes place in a wide range of healthcare institutions. Patients' blood is drawn for analysis in order to make diagnoses and track their health. Accurate and trustworthy results can only be achieved through the careful execution of defined protocols and the prioritization of patient safety and comfort.

Device selection, needle gauge sizes and lengths, evacuated tubes, order of draw, tube inversion, angle of insertion, quality control, tourniquet application and removal, skin integrity, venous sufficiency and contraindications, antiseptic agents and application, vein anchoring, problematic patients, potential complications, and adjustments during blood draw are all discussed in this chapter.

Medical personnel can reduce the risk of issues during blood collection and increase patient satisfaction by reading and understanding these guidelines.

For a successful blood draw, it is essential to use the proper blood collecting device. A hypodermic needle, which consists of a hollow cylindrical tube connected to a hub, is the most common tool used for routine blood collection. Needle gauge (diameter) and length are critical factors to think about before making a purchase.

There is a wide range of needle gauge sizes, from extremely fine (23G) to very coarse (18G). Patients with smaller veins or those needing smaller amounts of blood are better served by smaller gauge needles, while patients with larger veins or those needing larger volumes of blood are given needles with a larger gauge.

The depth of the intended vein and the patient's body size inform the choice of needle length. Needles typically range from 1 inch (25 mm) to 1.5 inches (38 mm), but those with fattier tissue may require a longer needle.

Blood samples are collected and transported in vacuum-sealed, sterile containers known as evacuated tubes. These vials can be found in a range of sizes, and their contents and drawing positions are indicated by color coding. Each container contains an additive designed to make some laboratory tests easier.

The order of draw specifies the order in which individual blood samples are drawn into individual, sterile, evacuated tubes. If you do things in the right order, you should get reliable test results. It may be necessary to invert the tubes gently after collection to ensure that the blood and additive are thoroughly mixed.

The angle at which a needle is placed into a patient's vein is known as the angle of insertion. Needle insertion angle is critical for optimum blood flow and minimal patient pain.

Needles, tubes, and other blood collection accessories should all undergo regular quality control inspections. This reduces the potential for contamination or malfunction during blood collection and helps maintain the equipment's integrity.

In order to see the veins and engorge them, a tourniquet is often placed around the patient's arm. Tight enough to restrict venous blood flow but loose enough to prevent arterial occlusion, it should be put 3 to 4 inches above the planned puncture site. Once blood flow has been restored, the tourniquet can be removed.

Finding a good vein for blood collection requires palpation, which is the examination of the patient's veins by touch. When deciding where to perform a venipuncture, a healthcare provider will employ palpation techniques to evaluate the vein's size, depth, resilience, and other characteristics.

A healthcare provider must first ensure the patient's skin is healthy and the chosen vein is strong enough to take blood from before beginning the procedure. A different location may need to be chosen if there are any skin lesions, infections, or scars in the area. The flexibility of the vein and the time it takes for the vein to refill after being compressed are used to determine the adequacy of the vein.

Complications can arise from collecting blood from a patient who has certain contraindications, such as an arteriovenous fistula or a location with a hematoma or infection.

Applying an effective antiseptic to the puncture site prior to venipuncture can help prevent the spread of infection. Isopropyl alcohol and chlorhexidine are two examples of alcohol-based antiseptics that see widespread use. Moving outward from the center, apply the antiseptic using a back-and-forth motion.

The healthcare provider must anchor the vein to stabilize it during venipuncture after locating the puncture site and prepping the skin. By doing so, the vein won't roll, and the blood draw will go smoothly.

Anxiety, obesity, dehydration, and problematic veins are just a few of the reasons why some people can be difficult to draw blood from. Healthcare providers can better adapt their methods and increase the likelihood of a successful blood draw if they have an understanding of the symptoms associated with these illnesses.

There is always a chance of something going wrong with a routine blood draw. Hematomas, phlebitis, nerve damage, fainting, and infections are all possible complications. Medical staff members need to be aware of these potential consequences, what may trigger them, and how to treat them.

Adjustments to the blood-drawing procedure may be necessary in some instances. Depending on the patient's health and individual needs, the needle's angle, needle gauge, or needle length may need to be modified.

Protecting healthcare workers against needlestick injuries and the spread of bloodborne pathogens requires the use of needle safety devices such as retractable or shielded needles. Use of these tools requires adherence to safety protocols.

Capillary blood collection is an alternative to venous blood collection in certain situations. The capillary bed of the skin is pricked with a lancet, and the blood is collected on special equipment. Similar to venous collection, the order of draw for capillary collection is based on the concept of least resistance.

Adhesive bandages or dressings made from sterile materials should be put to the puncture site after the blood has been drawn to promote hemostasis and stop any further bleeding. The bandage should be snug without restricting blood flow.

It is crucial to properly identify samples and preserve sample integrity throughout the laboratory testing procedure by marking blood collection tubes accurately. In addition to the collector's initials and the date and time of collection, the label should include the full name of the patient.

In conclusion, accurate and secure blood collection involves the use of established protocols and methods. Medical personnel can better ensure their patients' comfort and obtain high-quality blood samples for diagnostic testing if they have a firm grasp on all the details involved in the blood collection process.

Blood Collection Devices

Medical professionals often draw blood for testing and analysis, keeping tabs on patients, and conducting studies. Choosing the right blood collection device is essential for a smooth and effective venipuncture. Because of their direct effect on patient comfort, blood flow, and the quality of the collected sample, needle gauge sizes and lengths are crucial considerations in device selection. In this article, we'll talk in depth about the several types of blood collection devices, what goes into choosing one, and why needle gauge and length are so important.

Numerous blood collection technologies see regular use in healthcare institutions like clinics, hospitals, and labs. The hypodermic needle, a hollow cylindrical tube with a hub, is the most common tool used for routine blood collection. The hub allows for the attachment of ancillary tools like syringes and vacuum tubes. There are primarily three categories of blood collecting tools, including:

Needles, Typically Used

Most blood is collected with standard needles, also called straight needles.

They come in varying lengths and gauges to meet the needs of a wide range of patients and therapeutic applications.

Needles are typically simple in design, with a sharp beveled point used to pierce skin and get access to a vein.

Needles with wings, often known as butterfly needles:

Patients with small or frail veins, especially those who require numerous venipuncture attempts, can benefit greatly from the use of butterfly needles, also known as winged infusion sets.

They include little, bendable wings on one end that provide additional support and control during needle insertion.

The butterfly needle is attached to the syringe or other collection device at its opposite end.

Needles for Multiple Samples:

Needle sets with several evacuated tubes allow for multiple blood samples to be drawn without having to re-insert the needle.

A needle, adaptor, and tubing are the usual components.

When many blood samples are needed, these sets improve productivity by eliminating the need for multiple venipunctures.

Device Selection

To guarantee maximum patient comfort and a successful venipuncture, it is important to use the right blood collection device. Important things to think about include:

Types of Patients:

Depending on their age, people may need different gadgets. Butterfly needles, for instance, are frequently chosen by pediatricians.

The selection of a device is heavily influenced by the health and accessibility of the patient's veins. Needle sizes vary by vein size and fragility; smaller needles may be used for smaller veins.

Medical Requirements:

Device selection is affected by the volume of blood needed for analysis. When drawing a tiny amount of blood, a smaller gauge needle can be used, while a larger gauge needle is better suited.

Some laboratory tests have strict parameters for gauge size and blood volume for reliable findings. Selecting the right equipment requires consulting with lab personnel or referring to guidelines.

Needle Gauge Sizes and Lengths

When performing a venipuncture, the patient's comfort and blood flow are greatly influenced by the needle's gauge size and length. Typical needle gauges and lengths used for regular blood collection are described below.

Sizes of Needle Gauges:

There is a wide range of needle gauge sizes, from extremely fine (23G) to very coarse (18G).

Needles with lower diameters, as indicated by reduced gauge numbers, are used for knitting and crocheting.

Needles with a lower gauge have a smaller diameter, making them more appropriate for patients with weak veins, children, or when only a tiny amount of blood needs to be drawn.

Needles with a bigger gauge are used on patients with larger veins or when a greater volume of blood is required.

Distance Between Needles:

The length of the needle is also crucial when deciding on a tool.

The 1-inch (25 mm) and 1.5 inch (38 mm) needle lengths are the most often used for regular blood collection.

In individuals with an abundance of fat tissue or when the intended vein is situated deeper within the patient's arm, a longer needle may be required.

Needle gauge and length should be determined after carefully considering the patient's age, body mass index, vein health, and the volume of blood to be drawn. It is essential to strike a balance between patient convenience and vein accessibility while making these choices.

The specific needs of the laboratory tests and the planned use of the blood samples should also be taken into account by healthcare practitioners. In order to get reliable findings from some tests, certain gauge sizes or blood quantities may be required. Appropriate device selection is ensured by collaboration with laboratory professionals or by consulting established criteria.

Successful venipuncture relies on using the correct blood collection devices for routine blood collection. Medical facilities frequently make use of standard needles, butterfly needles, and needle sets designed to handle multiple samples at once. Patient characteristics, clinical demands, and laboratory requirements are only some of the variables that can affect which device is best.

Needle length and gauge size are two of the most important factors to consider while deciding on a device. However, bigger gauge needles are used for larger veins or larger blood pulls, whereas smaller gauge needles are utilized for frail veins or lesser blood volumes. The needle's length should be adjusted according to the patient's anatomy and the ease with which veins may be accessed.

Health care providers should prioritize patient comfort and safety during blood collection operations by carefully examining these aspects and selecting the most appropriate blood collection devices.

Evacuated Tubes

Blood samples are collected during venipuncture using evacuated tubes, which are sterile, vacuum-sealed containers. Different additives or anticoagulants are represented by different colours, and the tubes themselves come in a range of sizes. As soon as the needle is placed into the vein, the vacuum inside the tube begins drawing blood into it.

Order of Draw

When collecting blood, there is an optimal order in which various types of evacuated tubes should be filled. If you follow the steps in the right order, you won't have any problems with the test tubes becoming mixed up. The following is a common pattern for the order of the draw:

1. Collecting blood samples for microbial culture investigation can be done with the use of blood culture tubes. They have no additives and are completely sterile.

2. Prothrombin time (PT) and activated partial thromboplastin time (APTT) assays require the use of coagulation tubes, which contain anticoagulants like sodium citrate or EDTA.

3. Anticoagulants are not present in serum tubes, although clot activators or gel separators may be present. Liver function tests, lipid profiles, and kidney function tests are only

some of the biochemical tests that rely on them.

4. Arterial blood gas (ABG) analysis and some chemical studies require the use of heparin tubes, which contain the anticoagulant heparin.

5. Complete blood count (CBC), blood grouping, and blood typing all require the use of EDTA tubes, which contain the anticoagulant ethylenediaminetetraacetic acid (EDTA).

6. Additives in these tubes, such as sodium fluoride and potassium oxalate, prevent the breakdown of glucose in the blood, a process known as glycolysis. Fasting blood sugar and other tests that rely on precise glucose measurements employ these devices.

Sample contamination or influence from additives in the tubes can be avoided by drawing in the correct order.

Tube Inversion

After blood has been collected, the tubes containing any additives or anticoagulants should be inverted to ensure that the blood and additive are properly mixed. Inverting the tube can stop additives from clumping together or being distributed unevenly. The manufacturer's instructions and the type of tube you have will dictate the ideal number of inversions. The safety of the blood sample depends on your careful adherence to these procedures.

Angle of Insertion

Successful blood collection from a venipuncture relies heavily on the angle at which the needle is inserted. Vein depth, size, and condition all play a role in determining the optimal insertion angle, which is normally between 15 and 30 degrees. Superficial veins use gentler angles, but deeper veins may need more of a challenge. Successful venipuncture and minimal patient discomfort are both outcomes that are influenced by the angle at which the needle is inserted.

Equipment Quality Control

If you want trustworthy test results, you need to make sure the blood collection equipment is of high quality. There are many facets to this:

1. Always check for damage or faults before using a needle. Verify that the needles are clean and the packaging is unbroken before use. Needlestick injuries can be avoided by disposing of old needles in a safe manner.

2. Evacuated tubes should be inspected for damage and leaks before use. Discard any tubes that have been tampered with or exhibit evidence of contamination. Check the tubes' storage conditions and use-by dates.

3. Clean and well-maintained tourniquets are essential in an emergency. Tourniquets should be checked for damage and contamination on a regular basis. When using a tourniquet more than once, make sure to properly clean and disinfect it.

4. Syringes, adapter sets and extension tubing are examples of supplementary items; check that these, too, are sterile and in good working order.

Accurate test findings, contaminated samples, and patient injury can be avoided with regular equipment quality checks.

Tourniquet Application and Removal

During blood collection, tourniquets are used to briefly occlude veins, which increases venous engorgement and facilitates finding and accessing the vein. Patient safety and comfort depend on the tourniquet being applied and removed correctly.

How to Use a Tourniquet:

Choose a tourniquet size that allows you to securely wrap the patient's arm without applying too much pressure.

Make sure the tourniquet fits snugly and apply it 3–4 inches above where you plan to do the venipuncture.

Tighten the tourniquet until venous blood flow is reduced, but not so tightly that the patient is uncomfortable, or blood flow is compromised.

Release the Tourniquet

Once blood flow has been established and the needle is firmly inserted into the vein, the tourniquet can be removed.

When removing the tourniquet, do it gradually and smoothly so as not to interrupt blood flow.

To lessen the patient's discomfort and dizziness, explain how the tourniquet will be removed.

Patient comfort is increased, and problems like hematoma and venous stasis are less likely to occur, if the tourniquet is applied and removed correctly.

Palpation Techniques

A vein's suitability for venipuncture can be determined by a method called palpation. Locating veins and assessing their size, depth, and condition all need skilled palpation techniques. Vein palpation can make use of the following methods:

1. Check for visible veins by visually examining the patient's arm. Try to locate a large,

easily accessible vein for venipuncture.

2. Use the index and middle finger of one hand to hold the vein steady as you palpate it with the index finger of the other hand. This method is useful for determining the vein's size, depth, and strength.

3. Use moderate finger pressure and palpate in a systematic manner along the expected vein course to locate the best insertion site.

4. Use your fingers to apply pressure to a vein, then release the pressure and watch as the vein fills up. Vein health and adequacy can be evaluated with this method.

By using palpation techniques, medical professionals have a better chance of finding a safe insertion site and avoiding problems like unintentional artery puncture or a botched venipuncture.

Skin Integrity, Venous Sufficiency, and Contraindications Antiseptic Agents and Application Anchoring the Vein

Blood collection processes necessitate careful attention to the health of the donor's skin. The area where the venipuncture will take place should have healthy, unbroken skin that is free of any blemishes or illnesses. It's crucial to check for skin irregularities like cuts, bruising, rashes, and inflammation before the operation begins. It is critical to avoid further skin injury or infection by selecting a different venipuncture site if there are any damaged areas of skin. Additionally, special caution should be exercised to avoid areas of active inflammation or skin breakdown if the patient has disorders like dermatitis or eczema.

The term "venous sufficiency" describes whether or not the veins can hold enough blood after a venipuncture. Veins should be firm to the touch yet spring back after being compressed. Visible or palpable veins that fill and refill rapidly after pressure is released are indicators of venous sufficiency. Finding adequate veins for blood collection via palpation is one way to evaluate venous sufficiency. It may be necessary to use an alternative venipuncture location, such as the back of the hand or the forearm, if the veins are insufficient or difficult to access. Veins that are weak, sclerosed, or thrombosed should be avoided because venipuncture may fail or problems may arise.

Blood collection contraindications are any medical or personal history that makes venipuncture a bad idea. The existence of an arteriovenous fistula or graft (both of which are utilised in dialysis) is a common contraindication, as is the presence of an active infection or inflammation at the treatment site. Hematomas, bruises, and locations with a history of thrombosis or scarring at the desired site are also contraindications. Before collecting blood from a patient, it is important to get a full picture of the patient's health, medical history, and any specific reasons why blood collection shouldn't be done. If a vein cannot be punctured for whatever reason, capillary blood sample could be used instead.

The use of antiseptics is crucial for keeping the venipuncture site clean and free of infection. Antiseptics such chlorhexidine or isopropyl alcohol should be applied to the skin in accordance with the manufacturer's instructions prior to the procedure. It's important to wait until the antiseptic solution is totally dry before performing the venipuncture. Before inserting the needle, it is crucial not to contact the cleaned site or recontaminate it. Maintaining aseptic conditions during blood collection is essential to minimising the spread of disease and preventing the introduction of new organisms.

Vein anchoring is a technique used to prevent vein collapse or movement during venipuncture. Gentle traction on the surrounding skin or light pressure below the intended puncture location will suffice to anchor the needle. By using this method, the vein can be held in place during the needle insertion process for more precision. When anchoring the vein, care must be taken not to apply too much pressure or obstruct blood flow.

Blood collection from difficult patients may be complicated by their behaviour. There may be unique considerations and adjustments for these people due to their symptoms. Patients with needle phobia or extreme anxiety, for instance, may benefit from hearing reassurances and comforting words of encouragement. Patients with obesity or extra adipose tissue may need longer needles or other venipuncture sites because their veins are more difficult to access. Veins in the elderly can be more easily damaged, making them more susceptible to consequences like hematoma. Patient positioning and thorough monitoring during the procedure may be especially important for those with a history of fainting or syncope. In order to guarantee a positive blood collection experience for all patients, medical staff must be prepared to recognize the warning signals of difficult patients and respond accordingly. Protecting the donor's skin, making sure there are enough veins to draw from, and ruling out any potential complications are all crucial steps in the blood collection process. It is essential to preserve the patient's skin barrier at the venipuncture site to avoid infection and speed healing. Skin should be checked for wounds, blemishes, irritation, and infection before the operation begins. The risk of problems or future skin injury can be reduced by using a different venipuncture site if such abnormalities are present. Patients with dermatitis or eczema need more care because their skin is more likely to be sensitive and react negatively to treatments.

The term "venous sufficiency" describes how well the veins drain blood during a venipuncture. Feeling for veins that are perceptible, robust, and easily compressible is a frequent way to evaluate venous sufficiency by palpation. Adequate venous sufficiency is indicated by veins that are visible or palpable and quickly refill if pressure is released. Choosing veins that can carry the necessary blood volume without causing undue discomfort or difficulties is crucial. Avoiding venipuncture or experiencing bad reactions is important when dealing with veins that are fragile, sclerosed, or thrombosed.

Blood collection contraindications include everything that might make a venipuncture a bad idea or put the patient at risk. To avoid patient injury, it is important to thoroughly assess these warning signs. Common contraindications include places with ongoing infections or inflammation, areas with a dialysis-related arteriovenous fistula or graft, and sites with hematomas or bruising. Additionally, you should stay away from any spots where thrombosis or scarring have occurred in the past. Before performing a venipuncture, it is essential to have a thorough understanding of the patient's medical background, current health, and any potential complications. When venipuncture is not an option, capillary blood sampling can be used to obtain blood samples instead.

In order to avoid spreading infection at the venipuncture site, antiseptics are essential. The skin should be cleansed with an antiseptic before the procedure with either chlorhexidine or isopropyl alcohol. It's important to follow the instructions for using the antiseptic solution and wait for it to dry before attempting a venipuncture. Before inserting the needle, it is essential that no contamination be introduced by touching the cleaned area. Maintaining aseptic conditions during blood collection is essential to minimizing the spread of disease and preventing the introduction of new organisms.

The process of "anchoring the vein" is used to prevent the vein from moving or collapsing during venipuncture. Anchoring is done so that the vein does not move when the needle is being inserted. This can be accomplished by exerting light pressure below the desired puncture site or by gently tractioning the skin around the area. When anchoring the vein, care must be taken not to apply too much pressure or obstruct blood flow. The success rate of venipuncture can be increased, and patient discomfort can be reduced with proper anchoring each member of the healthcare team and the patient.

Problematic Patients: Signs and Symptoms

When discussing blood collection, the term "problematic patients" refers to people who may exhibit certain symptoms that make the process more complicated. Because of these symptoms, medical staff must take extra precautions, modify their procedures, and implement additional tactics to guarantee a successful blood draw.

Needle phobia or extreme anxiety is a prevalent problem. These individuals may experience extreme distress upon contemplating or being confronted with the prospect of a venipuncture. Symptoms of needle phobia include extreme panic, palpitations, perspiration, and even fainting. When dealing with such individuals, it is essential for healthcare providers to show compassion, patience, and understanding. The patient's anxiety and discomfort can be reduced by creating a soothing setting, explaining the operation in detail, and giving distractions or relaxation techniques.

Blood collection from patients who are overweight or have an abundance of adipose tissue might be difficult. Because of the additional fat, it may be more challenging to find and access veins. A

NHA Phlebotomy Study Guide

typical needle length may have difficulty reaching and palpating veins in these people. A longer needle or venipuncture locations like the back of the hand or the forearm, where veins may be more easily accessible, may be necessary in such instances. To avoid pain or other consequences, it's important to avoid pressing too hard on the area.

Blood collection from the elderly can be difficult due to variables such as weakened veins and less flexible skin. They may have a higher risk of experiencing a hematoma or an unsuccessful venipuncture because their veins are more likely to rupture or collapse during the process. These difficulties can be reduced by taking precautions such as touching the skin and veins gently, choosing proper venipuncture sites, and using appropriate needle diameters. In addition to making sure the patient is comfortable and safe, healthcare providers should keep a careful eye on them throughout the process.

It is important to take extra precautions while drawing blood from patients who have experienced fainting or syncope in the past. Anxiety, pain, or the sight of blood may cause these people to become lightheaded, dizzy, or even faint. Patients in this situation should be positioned such that they are lying down or sitting in a safe and comfortable position in case they feel dizzy and pass out. It is essential to keep the patient updated, reassure them, and continuously check their vitals throughout the surgery to ensure that no complications arise.

Patients with chronic diseases, vascular disorders, or impaired immune systems are also at risk for complications related to venous access. These patients' veins may be small or brittle, making venipuncture more difficult than usual. This may need the use of more sophisticated procedures, such ultrasound-guided venipuncture, or the exploration of other options, like capillary sampling or venous catheterization, for blood collection.

Possible Complications of Blood Draw

Even while drawing blood is usually risk-free, there are always chances for something to go wrong during or afterward. Healthcare providers must be alert to the potential for these problems and take measures to reduce their incidence. The following are examples of potential issues during a blood draw:

1. A hematoma is an extravascular collection of blood in a specific area. When a vein is ruptured or otherwise compromised during venipuncture, blood can seep out and cause tissue injury. Pain, swelling, and discoloration at the venipuncture site are all symptoms of a hematoma. Proper venipuncture practices, including providing light pressure after removing the needle, and ensuring appropriate hemostasis by exerting pressure and using a sterile gauze or bandage, can help prevent the formation of hematomas.

2. Vein inflammation, or phlebitis, can be caused by physical trauma, chemical trauma, or

an infection. It often presents as a red, heated, swollen, and painful vein. Aseptic procedures, careful vein selection, and a lack of unnecessary probing or friction can all help reduce the likelihood of phlebitis during blood collection. Phlebitis treatment may include anti-inflammatory drugs, warm compresses, and the elevation of the affected limb.

3. Rare but serious complications include infection at the venipuncture site. It is possible if the site is contaminated either before or after the surgery, hence it is important to use aseptic procedures. Inflammation, pus production, increased temperature, discomfort, and discharge are all symptoms of infection. Aseptic practices, safe disposal of used needles, and the use of appropriate antiseptics are all necessary to prevent infection when providing medical care.

4. **Nerve Injury:** If a nerve is accidently punctured or damaged by the needle during venipuncture, a nerve injury may result. The affected area may become numb, tingly, weak, or paralyzed as a result. Careful consideration of the venipuncture site, avoidance of sites with established nerve routes, and correct needle insertion procedures can all help reduce the likelihood of nerve injury. Immediate evaluation and referral to a specialist may be required if nerve damage is suspected.

Adjustments When Establishing Blood Draw

Adjustments may need to be made during the blood draw process to provide a smooth and safe procedure for the patient. The following are examples of possible modifications:

1. Healthcare providers may need to select a different venipuncture site if the one they initially chose is unsatisfactory or inaccessible. This may necessitate trying different veins on the same limb or switching to a new one. Considerations including vein visibility, palpability, size, and patient comfort should inform the choice.

2. **Needle Size and Insertion Angle:** The needle size and insertion angle may need to be modified based on the patient's age, body type, vein depth, and vein health. Patients who are overweight or have deeper veins may need longer needles to complete a venipuncture. Depending with the location and orientation of the vein, the insertion angle may also change.

3. Traditional venipuncture may not be an option or successful in obtaining blood in several situations. Capillary blood sampling and venous catheters are two alternatives to invasive jugular vein blood draws. Patients with problematic veins or those who need frequent blood drawing may benefit greatly from these techniques.

4. The success of the blood draw is highly dependent on the patient's position. Patients who

are at risk of fainting or syncope may benefit from lying down or reclined positions. Similar to how dangling the arm down or using a blood pressure cuff can enhance venous distension and make venipuncture easier, altering the arm posture can help.

Needle Safety Devices

Safe disposal of spent needles and prevention of needlestick injuries are primary goals of needle safety devices. These tools reduce needle reuse and safeguard healthcare workers from needlestick accidents thanks to built-in safety measures. Needlestick prevention tools include:

1. Needles that may be retracted into a sheath or shield are used in these instruments. When the needle is retracted into its sheath, it cannot cause an unintentional prick.

2. Safety Devices with a winged infusion set and a retractable needle are frequently utilised for blood collection from paediatric patients. Needles may be carefully retracted inside the device after usage, preventing accidental needlesticks.

3. After being removed from a patient's vein, the needle of a self-sheathing needle retracts into its sheath automatically. The withdrawal of the needle activates a mechanism that releases the sheath.

4. Needleless systems are those that don't require the use of needles to collect blood samples, instead relying on other methods such lancets or vacuum tubes with holders attached.

5. Accidental needlestick injuries are a leading cause of healthcare worker infection and other consequences; these accidents can be avoided with the help of needle safety equipment. If they are to be useful in encouraging safe blood collection practises, their use should be encouraged, and healthcare practitioners should be taught in their activation and disposal.

Capillary Collection (and Order)

Common sites for capillary collection include the fingertip and the heel, and the samples are often used for laboratory analysis. This is an excellent option when a venipuncture is not possible or when only a tiny amount of blood is needed for testing. First, a fingertip or heel is selected as an appropriate site for the treatment. You should pick a spot that has good blood flow and is devoid of any obvious lesions, scars, calluses, or cuts. After a location has been decided upon, the patient must be ready. Explain the procedure in detail to the patient and allay their anxiety. Reassure them that the treatment would be quick and painless to assist ease their nerves. The next step is to disinfect the area using an antiseptic solution, such as isopropyl alcohol or povidone-iodine, depending on the situation. The risk of infection can be minimised, and test findings can be trusted if the area is well cleaned. A sterile lancet is used to make a tiny hole in the skin after cleaning. The patient's age and the volume of blood to be drawn both affect the size of the lancet used. Adults should use a lancet with a gauge size of 21 to 23. Sterile gauze or cotton is used to clean away the initial bloodstain to prevent cross-contamination with other body fluids. Capillary tubes, microcontainers, or capillary collection devices are then used to collect further blood drops. Blood can flow more easily into the collecting device if the containers are held at an angle. The collected blood is then placed in the necessary test tubes or processed further. The suggested order of draw for capillary collection corresponds to the conventional venous order of draw and must be strictly adhered to. There will be less chance of contamination between tubes and more confidence in the results if you follow this order. Reliable and consistent capillary collection relies on proper technique and following the appropriate order of draw.

Bandaging Practices

Bandaging correctly after capillary collection is crucial for promoting healing, stopping bleeding, and lowering the risk of infection. After the blood sample has been taken, the puncture site is covered with a sterile gauze pad or cotton ball. Apply light, even pressure to the area to promote hemostasis and stop the bleeding. Tightness or pressure that restricts blood flow or causes discomfort should be avoided. After that, tape or another bandage wrap is used to keep the bandage in place. The bandage should be applied with caution so as not to restrict blood flow or cause pain to the patient. The cleanliness and integrity of the bandage should be examined on a regular basis. The puncture site should be checked for bleeding, edoema, or infection as soon as possible. An essential part of effective bandaging is educating the patient. The duration of any remaining bleeding, the need of keeping the puncture site clean and dry, and the need for immediate medical assistance in the event of problems should all be communicated to the patient. Bandaging correctly after capillary collection helps keep the patient comfortable and reduces the risk of infection.

Labeling Procedures and Considerations

Blood collection tubes must be clearly and accurately labelled to ensure patient safety, correct specimen identification, and accurate laboratory results. Tubes used to collect blood should be clearly labelled with pertinent information, including the patient's full name, a unique identifier (such as a date of birth or medical record number), the time and date of collection, and the initials of the healthcare provider who took the sample. During shipment, the labels shouldn't get smudged or fall off the tubes, and they should be easily readable. It is critical that labels adhere to any institutional rules or government regulations. Different sorts of tests may be given different colours of labels, and other information, including the doctor's contact info, may also be included. If a certain test needs to be labelled in a certain way or if electronic barcodes are being used to identify samples, medical personnel should be aware of this. Traceability and quality assurance in specimen handling and testing rely on accurate documentation of the labelling process. The reliability of laboratory testing relies on following proper labelling protocols and preventing the accidental mixing of specimens.

Chapter 7

Special Collections

The term "special collections" is used to describe the specialized methods and techniques employed during the gathering of diagnostic specimens. To get credible findings from these datasets, you need to have the right expertise. Some of the most often requested special collections are covered in this chapter. These include blood alcohol collection, blood smears, blood culture collections, pediatric volumes, throat cultures, nasal swabs, and nasopharyngeal (NP) culture swabs. We will also summarize the most important findings from these compiled works.

Smears of blood taken from the patient's periphery are prepared and examined under the microscope to provide a diagnosis. Red blood cells, white blood cells, and platelets are only some of the biological components of blood that may be learned about with the help of these smears. The process begins with drawing blood from a vein (a venipuncture) and ending with a drop of blood being distributed across a glass slide. Next, a spreading instrument or another slide is used to evenly distribute the blood. After the smear has dried, it will be colored so it can be viewed under a microscope. Blood problems like anemia, leukemia, and infections can often be diagnosed with the help of a smear taken from the patient's peripheral blood.

Microorganisms, and especially bacteria, can be detected in the circulation by blood culture collections. This method is essential for making a correct diagnosis of sepsis and pinpointing the exact infectious agent. Blood samples are collected from many places, most commonly via venipuncture, using aseptic methods to prevent contamination. The collected blood is placed into culture bottles equipped with growth material to foster microbial development. The bacteria in the culture bottles are given time to grow in a laboratory incubator. When healthcare providers get a positive culture result, they know they need to treat the patient with an antibiotic since bacteria or another germ is present.

The term "pediatric volumes" is used to describe the number of blood samples taken from young children. Due to their tiny stature, more delicate veins, and potential for increased discomfort or anxiety during blood collection, these individuals require special care and attention. Safe and effective blood collection requires the use of specialized equipment, such as lower gauge needles and blood collection tubes designed for children. When collecting blood from children, it is customary to take a smaller sample than would be taken from an adult patient of the same age and weight for the same set of tests. Pediatric blood collection can be a positive experience with the use of techniques including distraction, consoling measures, and parental involvement.

Collecting specimens from the respiratory system via throat cultures, nasal swabs, and nasopharyngeal (NP) culture swabs allows for the detection of bacterial and viral illnesses. During a throat culture, a swab is used to take a sample of the tonsils and pharynx from the back of the throat. Nasal swabs are used to acquire tissue samples from the nasal cavity. Culture swabs taken from the back of the throat are called nasopharyngeal (NP) swabs because they are taken by inserting a swab through the nose. Sterile swabs are used to collect these samples, which are then taken to a lab for further testing. In order to identify respiratory diseases including strep throat, influenza, and respiratory syncytial virus (RSV), doctors typically take swabs from the throat, nose, and nasopharynx.

Collecting blood samples for the purpose of determining alcohol content is known as "blood alcohol collection." Common applications include checking on people who are in rehab for alcoholism or who have been pulled over on suspicion of drunk driving. Blood alcohol testing is a reliable method of measuring a person's blood alcohol content, which can be used to evaluate impairment and monitor compliance with laws concerning the consumption of alcoholic beverages. Venipuncture is used to collect the blood, which is then sent for testing at a lab. If you want to get reliable findings from your samples, you need to follow the correct chain of custody rules.

In conclusion, special collections are a subset of diagnostic specimen collection using specialized methods and protocols. The morphology of blood cells can be studied and diagnosed with the help of peripheral blood smears. In order to diagnose infections in the bloodstream, blood culture samples are required. Blood collection from infants and children should be handled with extra care because of the high volumes involved. Nasal swabs, nasopharyngeal swabs, and throat cultures are used to diagnose respiratory infections. Forensic and medical objectives often necessitate the collection of blood for analysis of alcohol levels. Medical practitioners cannot provide correct diagnosis and care for their patients without first mastering the procedures and factors involved in specific collections.

Peripheral Blood Smears

Smears of blood taken from the patient's periphery are prepared and examined under the microscope to provide a diagnosis. Red blood cells, white blood cells, and platelets are only few of the blood's biological components that may be learned more about with this method. Haematological problems, including anemia, infections, and malignancies, can all be diagnosed and monitored with the help of peripheral blood smears.

Collecting a blood sample, usually via venipuncture, is the first step in completing a peripheral blood smear. A glass slide is then touched to the drop of blood, and the blood is transferred onto the slide. To uniformly distribute the blood, another slide is inserted at an angle of 30-45 degrees against the first slide and the two slides are pulled back and forth. This forms a uniform, single layer of blood cells on the glass slide. The smear is left out in the open to dry entirely.

Romanowsky-type stains, such as Wright's stain or Giemsa stain, are used to color the smear after it has dried. The stain reveals the unique morphological characteristics of the distinct blood cell types, making it easier to distinguish between them. Once the slide has been stained, it is viewed using both low and high magnification scopes.

The blood smear is examined under a microscope and scored on a number of different criteria. The size, shape, and distribution of red blood cells are studied. Different types of anemia and other blood disorders can be better understood through the lens of hematologic abnormalities such microcytosis (small cells), macrocytosis (big cells), poikilocytosis (abnormal shapes), and anisocytosis (changing cell sizes).

The size and shape of white blood cells are measured and compared to other cell types. Infections, inflammatory diseases, and leukemias can all be diagnosed with the use of a differential count, which measures the number of several types of white blood cells in the blood. Cells that aren't fully developed may be an indicator of disease.

Platelets are counted and examined for quality and quantity. Bleeding disorders and other platelet-related illnesses might be indicated by changes in platelet count or morphology.

The peripheral blood smear can reveal the presence of parasites like malaria parasites or microfilariae in addition to cellular components. These may be seen and studied in detail under a microscope to help doctors identify and characterize parasitic illnesses.

Professionalism and experience are essential for correctly interpreting a peripheral blood smear. Smear results are used in conjunction with other diagnostic tools and patient history to give a full picture of the patient's health. Flow cytometry and genetic analysis are two examples of more advanced diagnostic procedures that may be needed to characterize smear-detected abnormalities in further detail.

Blood Culture Collections

In order to identify microorganisms, typically bacteria, in the bloodstream, blood culture collections are necessary. This test is essential for diagnosing sepsis (blood infection) and identifying the offending pathogen, which directs subsequent antibiotic treatment.

Avoiding contamination during blood culture collection calls for strict adherence to aseptic technique. Collecting blood samples from multiple places is a standard part of the procedure. The probable infection source and the patient's state will dictate the collecting place.

The collection site is sterilized with an antiseptic solution like chlorhexidine or iodine before blood is taken. This aids in lowering the potential for pollutant introduction into the circulatory system. During the entire procedure, the doctor or nurse will keep their hands clean by wearing gloves and washing them frequently.

A blood sample is taken by inserting a sterile needle into a vein and transferring the blood into a blood culture container or vial. The amount of blood drawn is based on the patient's age as well as the lab's criteria. In order to increase the likelihood of identifying microorganisms, adult patients have their blood drawn and separated into two or more bottles (10-20 mL per culture set). The volume collected from children is proportional to their age and weight.

The needle is gently removed after blood is drawn, and the area is then compressed to encourage hemostasis. After the blood is drawn, it is moved to the correct blood culture bottles, where the collection time and location are carefully recorded.

The media in the blood culture bottles are designed to promote microbial growth. The bottles are then placed in an incubator set to conditions optimal for the growth of any microbes present. Signs of microbial development, such as increases in carbon dioxide or turbidity, are constantly monitored by automated blood culture equipment. When bacteria or other microbes are detected in a culture, the result is considered positive.

A pathogen's identity and antibiotic resistance can only be established once a positive culture has been confirmed through additional testing. This data is used to determine which antibiotic treatment is best in each individual case.

Rapid notification of the laboratory of a possible bloodstream infection is crucial for expedited processing of blood cultures. Patient outcomes can be improved through early intervention and tailored treatment made possible by timely reporting of positive results.

Pediatric Volumes

Due to their smaller stature, more delicate veins, and potential for increased discomfort or anxiety during the process, pediatric patients require additional care when blood samples are being obtained. When discussing the safe and comfortable collection of blood from infants and children for diagnostic purposes, the term "pediatric volumes" is often used.

Using lower gauge needles and blood collection tubes designed for children is an important part of collecting blood from children. When performing a venipuncture, utilizing a smaller gauge needle lessens the potential for trauma and suffering. Blood samples collected from children should be collected in pediatric-sized tubes to account for their age, weight, and the specific tests being performed.

When compared to adult patients, the amount of blood drawn from children is often smaller. Factors such as the child's age, weight, medical condition, and laboratory test requirements will determine the exact volume. Safe and effective blood collection from children requires strict adherence to established protocols and the advice of pediatric experts or laboratory personnel with competence in pediatric phlebotomy.

Distraction tactics can be used to help patients feel more at ease and experience less pain and anxiety throughout their procedures. For example, you could provide the kid with some age-appropriate entertainment like books, movies, or toys to play with. It can also be helpful to involve the child's parents or guardians in the operation and explain it to them in simple words.

It's common practice to choose the dorsal (back) surface of the hand or forearm as the venipuncture location. Veins suited for venipuncture are typically located in these regions because they are easily accessible. Vein size, visibility, and stability are all critical considerations when deciding where to insert the catheter in a child, but it is also crucial to do a thorough evaluation of the child's venous system. The selection of the vein for sample collection should prioritize the least intrusive method while still guaranteeing sufficient blood flow.

After deciding where to make the venipuncture, it's important to keep the child's nerves at bay by maintaining a soothing demeanor. When necessary, a kid should be restrained using proper procedures to protect both themselves and the healthcare provider. Distraction, mild immobilization, and the use of a parent or guardian to offer comfort and support are all techniques that have proven successful.

Alternative blood collection techniques may be used when venipuncture is difficult or impossible to perform. Capillary puncture is one such method, in which a small amount of blood is extracted by pricking the skin on a fingertip or heel. At the point of care, or in other situations where only a little amount of blood is needed, capillary blood collection is frequently employed. When performing a capillary puncture on a child, it is crucial to adhere to established protocols regarding the puncture site, depth, and collection tools.

The overall goal of pediatric blood collection is to collect precise and safe samples from young patients with as little discomfort and worry as possible. Healthcare providers must be prepared to adjust to the specific requirements of pediatric patients during blood collection by having the information, skills, and understanding to do so.

Throat Cultures, Nasal Swabs Nasopharyngeal (NP) Culture Swabs

Specimens from the respiratory tract are frequently collected using throat cultures, nasal swabs, and nasopharyngeal (NP) culture swabs in order to detect bacterial or viral illnesses. Strep throat, influenza, respiratory syncytial virus (RSV), and other respiratory illnesses can all be pinpointed with the help of these diagnostic techniques.

Samples of the tonsils and pharynx are taken from the back of the throat for throat cultures. The tonsils and back of the throat are swabbed using a sterile swab that has a soft tip. When collecting samples, it's important to keep your hands off the mouth and tongue. The swab is then sent to the lab in either a transport medium or a culture plate. Streptococcal pharyngitis (strep throat) is a bacterial infection typically caused by Streptococcus pyogenes, and it is diagnosed through a throat culture.

Swab samples are collected from the nasal cavity using nasal swabs. A sterile swab is inserted into one nostril and gently rotated against the nasal wall by the healthcare provider to collect nasal secretions. If necessary, the other nostril can be sampled using the same swab. When looking for respiratory viruses like influenza or respiratory syncytial virus (RSV), nasal swabs are often utilized.

Swabs taken from the back of the nose and the back of the throat are called nasopharyngeal (NP) culture swabs. The nasopharynx is reached by threading a flexible swab through the nostril. The secretions are gathered by rotating the swab against the nasopharyngeal wall. For example, germs like H. influenzae and Bordetella pertussis (whooping cough) can be detected with NP culture swabs.

It is critical to use good aseptic technique while taking samples for culture from the back of the throat, the nasal passages, or the NP. Using sterile swabs, staying away from non-sterile surfaces, and transporting specimens safely to the lab are all part of this process.

As soon as possible after collection, samples are sent to the lab to be processed and analyzed. Technicians in the lab either grow the samples in culture on the right medium or run them via molecular tests like polymerase chain reaction (PCR) to determine what kind of infections are present.

These diagnostic tests vary in their sensitivity and specificity based on a number of parameters, such as the severity of symptoms, the age of the patient, and the type of pathogens being tested for. Reliable and accurate outcomes necessitate proper training and adherence to standardized standards.

Blood Alcohol Collection

To determine how much alcohol is present in a person's blood, a blood alcohol collection is conducted. The forensic and legal communities frequently employ it in situations like workplace accidents and DUI investigations. The assessment of impairment and compliance with regulatory limitations relies heavily on the precision with which blood alcohol content (BAC) is measured.

Blood alcohol collection entails drawing a sample of a person's blood from a vein. To guarantee precision and a transparent chain of custody, the data collection process adheres to stringent protocols. The danger of contamination can be reduced if the individual taking the blood sample has been educated in phlebotomy skills and uses aseptic methods.

Antiseptic skin preparation of the collection site is the first step in the technique. To make finding and accessing the vein easier, a tourniquet may be inserted close to the site of collection. The size and gauge of the needle used depends on the patient's vein health and the volume of blood being drawn.

Once a vein is found, blood is extracted into a special vial or tube for testing blood alcohol content. There could be anticoagulants or preservatives in the vial to keep the sample from deteriorating. The collection tube must be clearly labelled with the patient's name, as well as the date and time the sample was taken.

After blood has been drawn, the incision is bandaged to prevent further bleeding and hasten the healing process. The acquired blood sample is carefully handled and sent off to the lab. Particularly in judicial proceedings, the integrity and traceability of the sample depend on strict adherence to chain of custody protocols.

The blood sample is analyzed using several methods in the lab to determine the exact alcohol levels. Detecting and quantifying alcohol content often requires gas chromatography or enzymatic tests. To provide precise and trustworthy outcomes, the lab employs standard operating procedures and quality control checks.

The removal of alcohol from the body causes a fluctuation in blood alcohol content. To get an accurate reading of the person's BAC, a blood sample should be taken as soon as possible after the alleged alcohol-related occurrence.

Key Takeaways of Special Collections

Getting accurate and trustworthy data from special collections such as peripheral blood smears, blood culture samples, and pediatric volumes calls for special approaches and considerations.

The morphology of blood cells can be gleaned from a peripheral blood smear, which helps clinicians diagnose hematological problems.

In order to identify bloodstream bacteria and direct effective antibiotic therapy, blood culture collections are crucial.

Blood samples taken from infants and children should be of a pediatric volume, which takes into account the patient's age, weight, and the number of tests that will be performed.

Specimens from the respiratory tract are collected by taking a throat culture, a nasal swab, or a nasopharyngeal (NP) culture swab to test for bacterial or viral illnesses.

Blood alcohol collection is the process of drawing blood from a vein in order to determine an individual's blood alcohol content.

Accurate diagnosis and effective patient management rely on proper collection techniques, adherence to aseptic procedures, and precise labeling in all special collections.

Specimens gathered for legal or forensic purposes require strict adherence to the chain of custody protocols to ensure their authenticity and traceability.

Healthcare providers and laboratory technicians must work together to ensure that obtained samples are handled, transported, and analyzed correctly during special collections.

In order to improve patient outcomes, it is crucial that the laboratory be informed of any suspicions or positive results as soon as possible.

Chapter 8

Dermal Puncture

I n order to collect blood samples for laboratory examination, dermal puncture (also known as capillary puncture or fingerstick) is commonly utilized. It's a helpful method for taking a small sample of blood from a vein in the finger or heel, where the capillaries are close to the surface of the skin. Dermal puncture is a viable alternative to venous blood collection in cases where only a small volume of blood is needed, in pediatric patients, or in patients with limited venous access.

The goal of dermal puncture is to get a sufficient blood sample while minimizing patient discomfort and the possibility of consequences. Dermal capillaries provide an abundant blood flow, enabling a reliable blood sample to be taken for medical diagnosis.

Choosing a good spot to make the puncture is a fundamental principle. Because of its convenience, the finger is often used as an injection site for adults. The index finger is sometimes used instead of the ring or middle finger. The heel is a common puncture location for young patients. The patient's age, body mass index (BMI), and the volume of blood needed for testing all play a role in determining the testing location.

Lancets, alcohol swabs, sterile gauze/cotton balls, and bandages/adhesive strips are all necessary for cutaneous penetration. The sharp needle or blade of a lancet is used to puncture the skin, and the item is discarded after usage. Depending on the age of the patient and the needs of the test, different sizes and gauges are available. Before the process, the puncture site is cleaned with alcohol swabs to prevent infection. After blood is drawn, the puncture site is compressed with sterile gauze or cotton balls to encourage clotting. After blood has been drawn, the puncture site is bandaged or covered with adhesive strips to prevent further bleeding.

Accurate and safe blood collection via dermal puncture necessitates a multi-step process.

Important steps in patient preparation include gaining informed consent from the patient after thoroughly detailing the operation. Checking for injuries, infections, or poor circulation at the puncture site are also crucial precautions to take before puncturing a patient.

The next step is to clean the area around the puncture location. To prevent infection and guarantee proper disinfection, an alcohol swab is used to wipe the puncture site. Make sure the puncture site is totally dry before proceeding.

Depending on the patient's age and the needs of the test, a different lancet size and gauge will need to be used for the actual puncture. After deciding where to make the puncture, the lancet is placed there, and the wound is formed quickly but carefully. How deeply the puncture is made is determined by the desired blood flow and the thickness of the patient's skin. After the lancet is withdrawn, blood flow is unrestricted.

A microcapillary tube or a collection strip are two examples of devices that can be used to collect blood. Accurate results from diagnostic tests depend on collecting a sufficient amount of blood for analysis. To avoid contaminating the tissue fluid, avoid milking or squeezing the puncture site excessively.

After the blood has been drawn, sterile gauze or cotton balls are used to apply mild pressure to the puncture site in order to encourage hemostasis. Once the bleeding has stopped, a bandage or adhesive strip is applied to seal the wound and prevent additional loss of blood.

Dermal puncture requires careful attention to a number of details. Children are particularly susceptible to skin damage since their skin is more fragile. When puncturing a baby or small child, it's best to do it in the heel, whereas older kids might be able to handle it in the finger. The pain and stress of pediatric patients can be lessened with the use of effective immobilization and distraction strategies.

The patient's medical history, especially diseases that may impact blood flow or clotting, should also be taken into account. Changes in capillary blood flow can impair the accuracy of a test in patients with circulatory diseases, edema, or reduced perfusion. When this happens, it may be necessary to look into other options for data collection.

The patient's age and skin condition should also guide the selection of a lancet size and gauge. Smaller, finer gauge lancets are needed to minimize trauma and pain in premature infants and neonates.

When venous access is difficult or only a little amount of blood is needed, cutaneous puncture is a useful technique for blood collection. Accurate and safe blood sample collection relies on medical practitioners having a firm grasp on dermal puncture's underlying concepts, necessary supplies, and standard operating procedure. It's important to take into account the patient's age, health background, and testing technique in order to keep the patient as comfortable as possible and provide the most accurate results possible.

Principles of Dermal Puncture

Capillary puncture, often known as a fingerstick, is a common method for collecting blood samples at the dermal (skin) level. Accurate and safe blood drawing requires medical personnel to have a firm grasp on the principles underlying cutaneous puncture.

Accessibility is an important consideration when performing a dermal puncture. It is crucial to choose a convenient location for blood collection to guarantee a smooth process. The finger is the most popular injection site in adults because it is easily accessible and has well-developed capillary beds. Since the ring and middle fingers have more surface area and more blood supply, they are commonly chosen. The index finger, however, can be substituted in its place. The heel is a typical choice for collecting capillary blood from pediatric patients. Choosing a puncture location that allows for sufficient blood flow and little patient discomfort is crucial.

The dermal puncture depth is another guiding principle. The piercing depth should be just right to ensure sufficient blood flow without causing damage to deeper structures. Considerations such as the patient's skin thickness and the needs of the test dictate the depth of the puncture. Finding the sweet spot between inflicting enough pain and tissue damage to get a good blood sample is crucial.

There are other rules for deciding where to make the puncture. The puncture location is chosen based on the patient's age, the reason for the test, and the patient's level of comfort. The adult fingertip's fleshy pad is typically used as a venipuncture site since it receives a good blood supply and is less sensitive than other regions of the body. Because of its increased surface area, the plantar surface of the heel is frequently utilized to draw blood from young patients. Choosing a good spot to puncture is essential for drawing a healthy blood sample.

Dermal puncture also relies on the notion of site rotation. To reduce the potential for tissue injury and discomfort, switching up where you get punctured is recommended. Minimizing tissue stress and the risk of consequences can be achieved by avoiding many punctures in the same region. To prevent contamination or buildup of substances that could skew data, it is best to switch up the puncture site on a regular basis.

Dermal Puncture Supplies

Having the right equipment is crucial for a successful cutaneous puncture treatment. The success of the surgery and the patient's comfort can be enhanced by careful supply selection and careful application.

Dermal puncture mostly relies on lancets as the supply of choice. A lancet is a single-use medical gadget that punctures the skin with a needle or blade. They are available in a wide range of diameters and gauges to meet the needs of a wide variety of patients and diagnostic procedures. Puncture success and minimal patient discomfort can be achieved by carefully selecting the appropriate lancet size and gauge. Pediatric lancets are made with smaller needles to lessen pain and prevent injury in young children.

Dermal puncture treatments also require the use of alcohol swabs. Before a procedure, they are used to remove debris, oils, and surface microorganisms from the puncture site. The potential for infection is thus diminished. Before puncturing, make sure the alcohol is entirely dry to avoid hurting or contaminating the blood sample.

After blood is drawn, it is pressed with sterile cotton balls or gauze to prevent bleeding. This aids hemostasis and stops any bleeding that could otherwise occur. To avoid the spread of infection and promote cleanliness, sterile gauze or cotton must be used.

After blood is drawn, the puncture site is covered with a bandage or adhesive strips. They keep the wound covered and assist stop bleeding while also soothing the sufferer. Keeping the puncture site sterile and encouraging healing requires the use of clean, correctly sized bandages or sticky strips.

When taking a blood sample via dermal puncture, a variety of collection devices can be employed. Common methods for collecting and transporting capillary blood to the proper laboratory tubes or containers for further investigation include the use of microcapillary tubes, micro collection containers, or collection strips.

Dermal Puncture Procedure

Dermal puncture is a method for collecting capillary blood samples for laboratory analysis. There is a specific protocol that must be followed for a successful blood draw.

1. Dermal puncture preparation involves informing the patient of what will happen and getting their permission to proceed. Make sure the patient is in a relaxed state and has everything they need before beginning the treatment. To prevent confusion or mistakes during data collection, proper patient identification must be verified.

2. Using soap and water or an alcohol-based hand sanitizer, the medical professional should wash their hands before beginning the treatment. This aids in keeping the area clean and safe from contamination.

3. Consider the patient's age, the test's intended use, and the patient's comfort level when deciding where to make the puncture. The fleshy pad of the fingertip is typically utilized by adults, but the heel is favored by many young patients. Select a place with adequate blood flow and stay away from swollen, scarred, or otherwise aberrant regions.

4. Remove any dirt, oils, or surface bacteria from the puncture site by wiping it with an alcohol swab. To achieve a complete cleaning, you should begin in the middle and work your way outward in a circular motion. To avoid any stinging or contamination of the blood sample, let the spot air dry completely.

5. Hold the lancet firmly and at a right angle (90 degrees) to the skin where you intend to penetrate. With consistent pressure, you can make a neat little hole in no time. Puncture depth should be adjusted based on patient age and skin thickness to ensure sufficient blood flow and minimise pain. Hemolysis and other tissue damage can occur if the puncture site is repeatedly squeezed or milked.

6. Once the puncture has been made, gentle, constant pressure should be applied to the surrounding tissue to stimulate blood flow and facilitate blood collection. Collect the capillary blood sample utilizing collection techniques like microcapillary tubes, micro collection containers, or collection strips. Carefully add the correct volume of liquid to the collection device.

7. After taking the blood sample, the lancet should be removed, and the puncture site should be bandaged with sterile gauze or cotton. This aids in the process of hemostasis, which stops bleeding. The creation of a clot depends on the pressure being applied for a sufficient length of time.

8. Once hemostasis has been achieved, the patient should be given the necessary care and comfort, and the procedure should be documented. Cover the puncture with a bandage or adhesive strip to keep it clean. Accurately record the procedure's start and end times, puncture sites, blood volumes, and any issues or observations that arose.

Special Considerations During Dermal Puncture

There are a number of factors that must be taken into account when performing a dermal puncture to guarantee the patient's well-being and reliable test findings.

Care must be taken to avoid injury when performing a dermal puncture on a child. In newborns and younger children, blood is typically drawn from the heel, whereas older children may be able to endure finger punctures. Effective immobilization and diversion methods are necessary for reducing stress and pain.

Sensitive skin, slowed capillary refill, and poor circulation are all issues that can affect the elderly. To prevent unnecessary trauma or skin rips, it is crucial to handle their skin with care. Choose a puncture site and gauge size carefully to reduce pain and maximize blood flow.

Prioritizing the patient's comfort during the dermal puncture technique is essential. Maintain open lines of communication with the patient, reassuring them and answering any questions or concerns they may have. Keep everyone as relaxed and comfortable as possible to lessen stress and discomfort.

Selecting a safe puncture site is especially important for patients with reduced circulation due to conditions like peripheral vascular disease or diabetes. Determine the state of the patient's blood vessels and stay away from them. The blood vessels can be widened and blood flow increased by applying heat to the puncture site prior to the surgery.

Controlling contamination and infections is essential for any skin puncture operation. Clean hands, hygienic equipment, and proper safety protocols are all part of this. After the puncture site has been cleaned, you should not contact it or any non-sterile surfaces.

The collection of capillary blood samples may be subject to test-specific restrictions. Learn the volume, collection procedure, and sample processing instructions for each test you plan to take. If you want reliable test results, you need to follow these guidelines.

Chapter 9

Newborn Screen

Public health initiatives that screen babies for certain genetic, metabolic, and congenital diseases are essential. Systematic testing of newborns is done to identify disorders that may not be obvious at birth but can have serious long-term health consequences if neglected. The objective, tests administered, procedures followed, the significance of early identification and intervention, ethical considerations, quality assurance measures, international perspectives, and future directions of newborn screening are all covered in this chapter.

The goal of newborn screenings is to detect diseases and conditions that can be effectively treated or controlled if caught at an early age. Disorders including phenylketonuria (PKU), congenital hypothyroidism, sickle cell disease, and cystic fibrosis are discussed in this chapter. Various newborn screening modalities, such as blood spots and hearing tests, are discussed, as well as the laboratory processes and techniques utilized to examine the samples. Integration of genetic and genomic techniques is just one example of a recent development in newborn screening that is highlighted in this chapter.

In order to fully appreciate the complexities involved in the early and precise detection of diseases in newborns, it is crucial to have a firm grip of the screening procedure itself. The need of screening at an early stage is emphasized in this chapter. Newborn screening sample collection, transport, laboratory testing, interpretation of results, and follow-up are all included. False-positive and false-negative results, as well as other difficulties, are discussed in this chapter.

Newborn screening is important because it allows for early discovery and treatment. The need of early diagnosis of problems in newborns to allow for early treatment and treatments is discussed. It discusses the potential difficulties in offering early interventions, the long-term advantages for affected persons, and the impact of early discovery on treatment outcomes. This chapter focuses on

NHA Phlebotomy Study Guide

how healthcare providers, parents, and the healthcare system can work together to improve outcomes for babies whose screenings come up positive.

Important ethical and legal concerns regarding the protection of individual rights and privacy are raised by newborn screening. Concerns about privacy, confidentiality, and parental rights in newborn screening are addressed in this chapter. It also discusses ethical concerns that may arise from newborn screening, including the sharing of information about a child's carrier status and the application of screening data to medical studies.

In order to get valid results from newborn screening, quality assurance and quality control must be strictly adhered to at all times. Quality control procedures for collecting samples, analyzing those samples, and reporting findings are discussed here. It discusses external quality assessment systems and proficiency testing that help laboratories evaluate their own results. The chapter also stresses the significance of ensuring that newborn screening laboratories are accredited and certified to ensure high quality.

The healthcare system, available resources, and cultural norms all play a role in shaping newborn screening programs. Different countries have different screening panels, policies, and techniques, which are discussed in this section. It also addresses international initiatives and partnerships that are working to standardize newborn screening protocols and facilitate the exchange of successful programs from around the world.

The chapter wraps up by looking ahead at where newborn screening is headed and what technologies are on the horizon. Possible future developments in newborn screening, including the use of genetic and genomic techniques, are discussed. Integration of newborn screening with precision medicine is also discussed in this chapter, as are developments that show promise for enhancing the accuracy and efficacy of newborn screening programs.

This chapter summarizes what is known about newborn screening and where it is headed in the future. Topics covered include why screening is done, what tests are given, how they are given, why early identification and intervention is so important, ethical considerations, quality assurance measures, international perspectives, and more. Healthcare providers, policymakers, and parents can all improve infant health outcomes by increasing the likelihood that problems will be detected and treated early on.

Newborn Screening Tests

Important diagnoses of genetic, metabolic, and congenital problems can be made by newborn screening testing. Conditions that aren't immediately apparent at birth but have serious consequences if untreated are the focus of these examinations. The tests included on the screening panel tend to change from country to country and healthcare system to healthcare system.

Phenylketonuria (PKU), congenital hypothyroidism, sickle cell anemia, cystic fibrosis, and hearing loss are only few of the common illnesses tested for in neonates.

Different approaches and procedures are utilized in newborn screening examinations. The collecting of blood spots via a heel prick soon after birth is one of the most prevalent ways. Markers or compounds in the blood are measured to determine the presence or absence of a condition. In addition, hearing tests can be used to check for hearing loss in infants. Improvements in newborn screening technology, such as the incorporation of genetic and genomic techniques, have been made throughout the years. These developments permit for more thorough and precise screening, which in turn increases detection rates and permits for early interventions.

Process of Newborn Screening

Several procedures are used in newborn screening to guarantee early and accurate diagnosis of diseases. Most screenings are performed within the first 24 to 48 hours following delivery, which is when the screening timetable begins. The first step is sample collection, which commonly entails a heel prick to draw blood. Some diagnostic procedures may call for an extra specimen, such as urine or saliva.

After samples have been gathered, they are sent to a lab for further examination. The indicators or compounds associated with the screening disorders are measured using a variety of laboratory techniques and methodologies. Depending on the screened-for condition, the analysis could employ enzymatic assays, immunoassays, molecular genetic testing, or other niche methods.

The screening results must be interpreted before proceeding. To determine whether a newborn has a positive or negative screening result, laboratories will compare the measured levels to predetermined cutoffs or reference ranges. Keep in mind that a positive result just suggests the need for additional diagnostic testing, not that the problem is really present.

Procedures for reporting and following up on newborn screening results are crucial. Healthcare practitioners tell parents or guardians and propose additional diagnostic testing if a newborn obtains a positive screening result. Timely interventions and adequate follow-up care depend on early communication and coordination among primary care physicians, parents, and specialists.

Importance of Early Detection and Intervention

The success of newborn screening programs depends on their ability to detect and treat problems early on. The fundamental objective of newborn screening is to detect illnesses at their earliest stages, when they are most treatable and can have the greatest impact on health outcomes. The earlier a health problem is identified, the more likely it is that it can be treated, halted, or at least mitigated.

If caught early enough, several illnesses can be treated effectively before they cause death or permanent disability. A good example is the genetic disorder phenylketonuria (PKU), which can be detected through neonatal screening and treated with a particular diet to keep afflicted infants healthy.

Early detection and action not only prevent negative health consequences, but also reduces healthcare costs. Treating diseases in their early stages is typically more successful and less expensive than treating them in their later, more advanced stages.

Additionally, genetic counseling and informed family planning are made possible by newborn screening. Parents of affected infants will have a greater understanding of the condition and its potential long-term effects and will be better equipped to make decisions about family planning and resource acquisition.

Ethical and Legal Considerations

To preserve individual rights, privacy, and the proper use of screening data, ethical and legal questions take center stage in the context of neonatal screening. There are several major moral and legal considerations:

Newborn screening is important, but it must be done with careful attention to informed consent and parental rights. While screening is routinely done, it is always important to get parental permission before proceeding with any tests. Parents have the right to refuse or accept screening, and they should be given explicit information about the reasons for doing either. The freedom of choice and the authority of parents must be respected.

Data collected during newborn screening must be kept private and confidential to protect the privacy of families. During both the first screening and any later follow-up treatments, it is crucial that the privacy of both the newborn and their family be protected. Screening findings and associated data should be retained safely, accessible only by authorized personnel, and used just for healthcare purposes, thus it's important to take precautions to prevent their misuse.

Another important ethical factor is whether or not to reveal one's carrier status. Even if a newborn shows no signs of a genetic disorder, knowing whether or not the mother is a carrier can affect how they choose to expand their family in the future. In order to help parents make educated decisions about their reproductive options, proper carrier disclosure necessitates offering them with correct information, adequate counseling, and support.

Incidental discoveries, which are sometimes discovered during newborn screening, can present ethical challenges. The term "incidental findings" is used to describe the detection of diseases or genetic variants that were not originally planned to be found during the screening process. The clinical relevance, available therapies, and potential advantages or harms to the child and family must all be carefully considered before making decisions regarding reporting and acting upon incidental findings.

Quality Assurance and Quality Control in Newborn Screening

Measures of quality assurance and quality control are essential in newborn screening to guarantee effective screening and accurate outcomes. The following are essential features of quality assurance and control:

The gathering of samples is the first step in quality control procedures. To avoid compromising the quality of the samples, correct collection methods and defined protocols must be followed. Sample collection errors can be reduced, and consistency can be preserved by training and educating the healthcare personnel who handle them.

Quality assurance procedures in a laboratory are essential for producing trustworthy results. To do this, laboratories must adopt standardized protocols, calibrate their instruments, validate their testing procedures, and take part in proficiency testing. The precision and dependability of laboratory procedures can be monitored and preserved by consistent internal quality control checks and adherence to external quality evaluation programs.

Quality control measures for newborn screening tests should always include accreditation and certification of testing facilities. Labs that demonstrate expertise in their testing techniques, a commitment to continuous quality improvement, and a dedication to best practices are all characteristics of laboratories that have earned accreditation. However, certification programs offer further verification of laboratory expertise and adherence to guidelines.

The screening program needs constant inspection and monitoring to pinpoint problem areas and keep quality high. Audits, data analyses, and feedback loops can find problems in the screening process before they become major. These procedures allow for immediate action to be done, when necessary, which improves quality control and assurance in newborn screening as a whole.

International Perspectives on Newborn Screening

Different countries have different newborn screening programs due to differences in healthcare infrastructure, available funds, cultural norms, and the prevalence of diseases. Newborn screening from a global perspective involves many factors:

There are regional and national variations in newborn screening panels. Disease prevalence, treatment options, and access to medical care are only a few of the variables that affect which illnesses are included in national screening panels. Because of these differences, it is essential that newborn screening programs be adapted to meet the requirements of each individual country or region.

The rules and regulations of screening also vary from one nation to the next. Each nation sets its own regulations and recommendations for newborn screening, including the conditions that should be screened for, when screening should occur, and how it should be performed. The enhancement of screening programs around the world is facilitated by international collaboration and the sharing of best practices.

Newborn screening faces a variety of obstacles and possibilities depending on where it is implemented. It may be difficult for low-income nations to launch and maintain robust newborn screening programs. However, with the right supervision, technical assistance, and capacity building, international collaborations and partnerships can help overcome these obstacles. Newborn screening programs can be improved globally through the exchange of information and experiences between countries.

Future Directions and Emerging Technologies

The development of new tools and a deeper comprehension of genetic and metabolic abnormalities have pushed newborn screening forward. Some potential developments and new tools in neonatal screening are:

The addition of novel illnesses to newborn screening panels. New illnesses that might respond to early diagnosis and treatment are being discovered all the time as science progresses. As more research is conducted and new treatments are introduced, it is possible that newborn screening panels will be expanded to include additional disorders.

Newborn screening using an integrated genetic and genomics approach. More thorough and accurate screening may be possible with the help of genetic and genomic technology. Newborn screening can be made more precise and time-efficient with the use of modern technologies like next-generation sequencing (NGS), which enables the screening for numerous genetic disorders at once.

Premature infant screening combined with targeted therapy. The goal of precision medicine is to personalize patient care by taking into account their specific genetic makeup and environmental factors. Health outcomes can be improved by integrating newborn screening with precision medicine approaches, which can lead to individualized interventions and therapies for each newborn.

Developments in the fields of data administration and informatics. Because of the volume of data produced by newborn screening, advances in data administration, analysis, and informatics are needed. Improve the efficiency of newborn screening programs by employing AI and machine learning algorithms to aid in data interpretation, risk prediction, and decision support.

Chapter 10

Processing

Important steps are taken during processing to guarantee reliable specimen handling and testing, making it a critical step in the laboratory workflow. Chain of custody, key values for point-of-care testing, and the dissemination of results are only some of the topics covered in this chapter, along with centrifuging, aliquoting, handling, storing, transporting, and disposing of specimens. These critical steps are essential to the laboratory's capacity to offer accurate and timely diagnostic results to doctors and other medical professionals.

In the laboratory, centrifugation is frequently employed for density-based separation. Denser components, such as cells or particles, sink to the bottom of the tube during rapid rotation, while lighter components, such as serum or plasma, rise to the top. Some diagnostic procedures, like blood chemistry and microbiological cultures, require extremely small sample volumes, making centrifugation an absolute necessity. Accurate results can only be obtained with careful centrifugation, as improper separation can lead to incorrect interpretations and poor patient care.

Aliquoting is used after centrifugation has been completed. To aliquot a specimen is to divide it into smaller, more manageable pieces that can then be tested, stored, or transported with ease. The integrity of the original sample is maintained while the laboratory gets access to a sufficient amount of material for testing thanks to careful aliquoting. Using the right containers and labelling methods is crucial for avoiding contamination and keeping track of everything.

During the processing phase, specimens are handled, stored, transported, and disposed of. Avoiding mistakes and preserving the quality of samples requires the use of proper handling practices such labelling, documenting, and adherence to safety protocols. Specific conditions, including temperature and light exposure, must be met in order to keep samples stable throughout storage. Furthermore, specimens must be packaged appropriately and transported from collection sites to the laboratory in accordance with standards to prevent damage or degradation. Finally, in order to reduce hazards to people and the environment, specimens, including biohazardous materials, must be disposed of in accordance with approved guidelines.

Forensic and legal processing relies heavily on the concept of the chain of custody. This term is used to describe the paper trail left behind by the collecting, storage, and delivery of specimens. The integrity and admissibility of test results as evidence in judicial proceedings depend on the maintenance of a safe and reliable chain of custody. In order to ensure the integrity of the results and keep people's faith in the laboratory's abilities, strict protocols and documentation must be adhered to in order to prevent the manipulation, loss, or contamination of specimens.

Critical values play a crucial role in patient management and immediate action in point-of-care testing (POCT). A critical value is a diagnostic threshold at which emergency medical care is required. Medical providers need timely notification of crucial value thresholds established by laboratories. Timely clinical decision making, and proper patient care rely on the prompt and correct reporting of essential values.

When the results are disseminated, processing is complete. Test results must be communicated to healthcare practitioners as soon as possible, and the laboratory is responsible for making sure that this happens in a safe and timely manner. This is where things like laboratory information systems or electronic health record systems come in handy, since they streamline communication, reduce the likelihood of mistakes, and improve the efficiency with which results are reported.

Centrifuging

Separating parts of a material based on their densities by means of centrifugation is a fundamental laboratory technique. High-velocity rotation of the specimen creates centrifugal force, which separates the denser components from the lighter ones, sending the former to the bottom of the tube and the latter to the top. The fields of clinical chemistry, hematology, immunology, and microbiology, to name a few, all make extensive use of centrifugation in their lab work.

Centrifugation's main function is to separate out target diagnostic sample types. The cellular components of blood, including red blood cells, white blood cells, and platelets, can be separated from the liquid plasma or serum by centrifugation. This separation is essential for the correct interpretation of laboratory investigations such as blood chemistry tests and coagulation studies.

There are a number of considerations that need to be made in order to have successful centrifugation. First and foremost, it's crucial to use a centrifuge and rotor that are well-suited to the task at hand. There are several variations of centrifuges, each with their own unique capacity and maximum speed, such as ultracentrifuges, high-speed centrifuges, and tabletop centrifuges. The volume and nature of the specimen dictate the rotor that must be used for centrifugation. Each centrifuge and rotor comes with its own set of instructions and requirements that must be met for the machine to function properly and safely.

Choosing the appropriate centrifuge speed, or relative centrifugal force (RCF), is also crucial. Separation efficiencies vary depending on the specimen type, hence RCF is typically stated as a multiple of gravity (g). Careful consideration of the specimen's properties and the intended use of the test should guide the choice of centrifugation speed and duration. Improper centrifugation can harm samples or cause hemolysis if done for too long, while insufficient centrifugation can lead to incomplete separation and false results.

It is also important to handle specimens correctly before and after centrifugation. Labelling specimens correctly is crucial for proper identification and can help with tracking. Under or overfilling tubes can have a negative impact on the separation process and should be avoided. In addition, centrifugation safety requires that tubes be securely closed to prevent leakage or aerosol production.

Without disturbing the settled portion, the separated components should be carefully removed during centrifugation. Pipettes, precise decanting, and automated techniques are commonly used for this purpose. Maintaining the purity of each fraction and preventing contamination between them is essential. Cells and microbes are examples of delicate components that require special treatment to avoid damaging or disrupting their structures.

Aliquoting

The term "aliquoting" refers to the process of cutting a sample into smaller, more manageable pieces. Multiple tests, long-term storage, and portability are just some of the many applications for aliquots. Aliquoting is an essential part of the laboratory process since it guarantees that sufficient specimen is available for examination without jeopardizing the original sample.

Aliquoting is done so that the specimen can be divided into smaller portions that can be used for a variety of tests in the lab. Aliquoting a blood sample for separate tests like glucose, electrolytes, liver function, and kidney function is one common practice when collecting samples for a metabolic panel. This eliminates the need for several blood draws and reduces patient discomfort as well as the possibility of human mistake by performing multiple tests on the same specimen.

Laboratory specimens must be aliquoted correctly to ensure their correctness and traceability. The first step is to find suitable aliquot containers. The aliquoting containers must be clean, leak-proof, and appropriate for the specimen. Aliquots of urine, for instance, may need to be maintained in special containers containing preservatives to ensure sample stability, while aliquots of serum or plasma are commonly stored in cryogenic vials or screw-top tubes.

The utmost care must be taken while aliquoting to avoid both intra- and inter-aliquot contamination. This is accomplished by utilizing aliquoting instruments that are specific to each specimen, such as disposable pipettes or automated aliquoting devices. Using disposable equipment reduces the time spent cleaning and disinfecting between aliquoting stages and eliminates the possibility of cross-contamination.

To guarantee adequate identification and traceability throughout the laboratory workflow, accurate labelling of aliquots is essential. Patients' names, specimen types, test dates, and other identifying information should be accurately labelled on each aliquot. The use of barcode labels or other forms of unique identification can also help automate tracking and lessen the potential for human mistake in follow-up testing and reporting.

When storing specimens, aliquoting is also an important step. Aliquoting is a method for preserving specimens for later testing or archiving without jeopardizing the integrity of the original sample. To keep samples from degrading during storage, factors like temperature, light exposure, and length must be taken into account.

Aliquoting is necessary for transporting specimens, as well as for testing and storing them. The potential for specimens to be damaged or leak during transport is lessened if they are aliquoted into smaller amounts. Aliquot containers that have been properly sealed and labelled can withstand transportation stresses and reduce the likelihood of sample loss or tampering.

The laboratory processing stage is not complete without the use of centrifugation and aliquoting. Using centrifugation, components of a material can be separated based on their density, allowing for more precise diagnostics. But aliquoting lets you divide samples up into smaller portions for easier handling, storage, and transport. Laboratory testing contributes to the quality of patient care when it is performed with integrity, accuracy, and efficiency thanks to standardized processes for centrifugation and aliquoting.

Handling, Storage, Transportation, and Disposal of Specimens Chain of Custody

The integrity, safety, and traceability of specimens from collection to final disposition depend on the proper handling, storage, transportation, and disposal of specimens throughout the laboratory process. To keep specimen quality high and laboratory results trustworthy, it is crucial to adhere to standardized protocols and best practices in these areas.

Correct specimen handling starts with the collection process. It requires paying close attention to the collecting procedure, such as by utilizing suitable containers, adhering to aseptic practices, and making sure everything is properly labelled and documented. Care should be taken when handling specimens to prevent any potential for contamination, deterioration, or loss of integrity. Workers in laboratories should be educated on how to safely handle potentially infectious or hazardous items and required to follow all relevant safety measures.

The safety of the patient and carers must always come first during any kind of handling. When dealing with potentially infectious or biohazardous specimens, it is important to use appropriate personal protective equipment (PPE) such as gloves, lab coats, and face masks. As an added precaution against exposure or environmental contamination, any spills or accidents should be dealt with immediately in accordance with established guidelines.

It is crucial to properly store specimens to keep them stable and undamaged until testing can be done. To maintain their qualities and prevent deterioration, different types of specimens call for specialized storage environments. The specimen type and test needs will determine how temperature, humidity, and light exposure should be managed.

Specimens like blood, urine, and tissue samples need to be kept at a cool temperature, hence refrigerators and freezers are frequently employed for this purpose. To ensure the units stay within the specified temperature range, they should be checked and calibrated frequently. Specialized storage conditions, such as controlled atmospheres or specialized growth media, may be necessary for some specimens, such as volatile analytes or certain microbiological cultures.

It is essential that specimens be properly labelled and organized in storage for easy retrieval and tracking purposes. The patient's name, the date of collection, and any other identifying information should be clearly labelled on each specimen. Laboratory information management systems (LIMS), often known as specimen tracking systems, help keep tabs on and retrieve stored samples with ease and accuracy.

Sample integrity and prompt processing rely on the transit of specimens from collection sites to the laboratory. All participants, including couriers, healthcare practitioners, and laboratory staff, need to be aware of and follow established transportation protocols.

Transporting specimens requires a leak-proof container that is properly labelled. Additional protection and temperature control during transport may necessitate the use of secondary packing like biohazard bags or insulated coolers. It is critical to adhere to safety standards and prevent potential dangers by following legislation and recommendations for the transportation of hazardous materials, especially biohazardous specimens.

Those responsible for transporting packages or other items should be educated on safe handling practices and given detailed instructions on how to do so. Specimens that must be kept within a certain temperature range during transport may benefit from the usage of monitoring equipment like temperature loggers.

When talking about specimens, the term "chain of custody" refers to the paper trail that follows them from the point of collection to wherever they end up. When specimens are utilized as evidence in a forensic or legal setting, this is of paramount importance. The integrity and admissibility of laboratory results can be safeguarded against tampering, loss, or contamination with the help of a secure and dependable chain of custody.

Several important factors must be in place for a chain of custody to be set up and kept in good standing. These include clear labelling and sealing of specimens at each stage, identification of all personnel involved in handling the specimen, and precise and full documentation of specimen collection. There should be a signed receipt or transfer of custody document from each person who handles the specimen.

Strict standards must be followed in forensic or legal situations to ensure the chain of custody is kept and can be used as evidence. For example, you may use tamper-evident seals, keep the storage area locked down, and record any incidents that occur while you're working with the specimen.

It is critical that specimens and other laboratory waste be disposed of properly in order to avoid contaminating the environment, ensure the safety of laboratory workers, and meet applicable rules and requirements. Specimens, biohazardous materials, and other laboratory waste should be disposed of in accordance with established policies and procedures.

Separating specimens and other hazardous materials from the laboratory waste is important. Disposal of biohazardous waste should follow regional guidelines and may involve autoclaving, chemical treatment, or incineration. Standard waste management practices call for the proper recycling or disposal of non-hazardous trash, such as discarded specimen containers and packaging materials.

Accurate records of waste disposal activities, including waste kind, quantity, disposal method, and necessary permits or approvals, should be kept by laboratories. Compliance with waste management regulations may be ensured and improvement areas can be found through routine audits and inspections.

Correct specimen management includes collecting, preserving, transporting, and disposing of samples. Standardized methods and best practices in these areas assist safeguard the safety of employees and the environment, help keep specimens intact and traceable, and provide credibility to laboratory findings.

Critical Values for Point of Care Testing

Diagnostic testing that is conducted away from a centralized laboratory but still close to the patient is called point of care testing (POCT). The quick turnaround time of these tests allows doctors to act quickly on patient diagnoses. When a point-of-care test (POCT) reveals a critical value, it means the patient needs emergency medical care.

Setting cutoff levels for POCT is important for early detection and treatment of serious problems. Factors such as the analyte being measured, the patient demographic, clinical recommendations, and the severity of the issue must all be taken into account when establishing critical levels. Different tests, facilities, and patient populations can result in different critical values.

Laboratory experts, healthcare providers, and other key stakeholders work together as part of a rigorous process to determine critical values. In doing so, it may be helpful to examine legal regulations and professional recommendations, as well as to consult with clinical professionals and analyze past significant occurrences.

All relevant healthcare workers should have ready access to the determined important values, which should be meticulously documented, widely disseminated, and readily available. They could be published as part of a crucial results log or report, or they could be included in a laboratory's reference ranges. In addition, laboratories should have well-defined rules and processes in place for the early dissemination of essential values to healthcare professionals.

Important values should be transmitted in a consistent, trustworthy, and documented manner. When alerting medical professionals, laboratories frequently resort to tried-and-true means including phone calls, encrypted message systems, and notifications via electronic health records. Confirmation of identity, receipt, and comprehension of the critical value should all be part of the communication process. For both legal and quality assurance reasons, it is crucial that the communication be recorded.

When a critical value is reported, medical staff members should act in accordance with established guidelines. This may entail contacting the patient, beginning urgent therapy or intervention, notifying the appropriate clinical teams, or calling for emergency assistance. Actions made in response to essential values should be documented by healthcare professionals to ensure continuity of care and accountability.

Monitoring and assessing the treatment of critical values in POCT requires quality assurance programmes. Critical value reporting entails continuous monitoring, tracking of reaction times, evaluation of intervention appropriateness, and investigation of adverse occurrences and near-misses. Activities like these aid in spotting trouble spots, guaranteeing adherence to rules, and boosting patient security.

When it comes to diagnosing potentially fatal illnesses at the point of care, key values are indispensable. Patient safety and the provision of timely, high-quality healthcare are aided by the establishment of clear and suitable critical values, the implementation of effective communication systems, and the verification of acceptable clinical activities.

Distribute Results

Communicating test results to the right healthcare practitioners or authorized personnel is an essential part of the laboratory process that plays a crucial role in patient care. Timely decisions, continuity of treatment, and clear lines of communication between the laboratory and healthcare teams all depend on prompt and correct delivery of results.

Laboratory capabilities, test types, and the availability of communication infrastructure are all factors that might affect how results are disseminated. Nonetheless, there are a few common factors to keep in mind for efficient outcome distribution:

It is important to double check test results for accuracy and completeness before releasing them to the public. The right patient ID, test name, and measurement units must all be verified. Results can be trusted since they have been subjected to quality control techniques and reviewed by trained laboratory specialists.

Methods of Dissemination: Whether electronic, by fax or other secure messaging platforms, or in the form of printed reports, the results can be disseminated in a number of different ways. The transmission of laboratory findings should occur via trusted and secure methods to ensure patient privacy and adherence to applicable data protection laws. The distribution of test results is simplified, and transcription errors are minimized thanks to electronic connections between the laboratory information system (LIS) and electronic health records (EHRs).

Healthcare providers frequently need to interpret laboratory data in order to use them to guide patient management. Reference ranges, interpretive remarks, and clinical decision support tools are all examples of what laboratories should provide to help doctors use their findings correctly. This ensures that data are correctly interpreted and allows for more well-informed clinical decisions to be made.

Prioritizing Results Laboratories should develop systems to identify and highlight urgent or abnormal test results. As was said before, results such as critical values warrant immediate communication. Laboratories facilitate fast action by healthcare professionals by clearly recognizing and indicating these results, reducing the potential for delays in crucial patient treatment.

Timeliness of reporting is essential for effective patient care. It is important for labs to set turnaround time goals for various tests and regularly meet them. The time it takes to report results has decreased thanks to the implementation of automated systems, real-time notifications, and optimized workflows. Quality assurance and finding places to improve rely heavily on monitoring and reporting turnaround times.

It is crucial that test results be made available to authorized personnel involved in patient care. Access to laboratory results should be governed by well-defined policies and procedures, with appropriate authentication and role-based controls in place. Healthcare providers and patients benefit from increased engagement and collaborative decision-making when they have easy, secure access to results through web portals, electronic health record integration, or patient portals.

For legal, regulatory, and quality assurance purposes, it is crucial to maintain accurate records of all activities related to disseminating results. It is important for laboratories to keep detailed records of all communications and actions related to the distribution of results. If there are any questions or concerns about the dissemination of results, this record can be used to trace their origin, verify their accuracy, and investigate the problem.

By paying attention to these factors, labs can improve the coordination of patient care and the quality of communication between the lab and healthcare professionals.

Key Takeaways of Processing

Accurate and trustworthy test findings depend on the thoroughness of the laboratory's specimen-processing procedures. Separating a specimen's components based on their densities, which centrifugation does, is crucial. High-speed spinning separates the specimen's denser components, enabling for the separation of the analyte of interest and the elimination of any interfering compounds. Correct centrifugation settings are essential for preventing specimen hemolysis and other unwanted side effects.

The procedure of dividing specimens into smaller sections, known as aliquots, is also crucial to the processing phase. This is necessary for numerous types of testing, as well as storage and transit. The original specimen is less likely to be tainted or degraded when aliquots are used. Aliquots must be properly labelled with patient information and other identifiers to allow for easy identification and traceability at every stage of testing.

Important factors in processing include care in handling, storage, transport, and disposal of specimens. Careful handling of specimens necessitates adherence to recognized safety measures and the use of suitable PPE. For specimens to remain stable and undamaged, appropriate storage conditions, including temperature regulation and labelling, must be maintained. Transporting samples without losing or compromising them requires secure packaging, compliance with standards, and adequate tracking. The proper disposal of specimens and other laboratory waste is essential for the protection of human health and the environment.

Tracing and documenting specimens from collection to final disposition—known as the "chain of custody"—is an essential part of specimen processing. This is especially important in forensic and judicial settings to assure the reliability of laboratory results. Maintaining the chain of custody and ensuring traceability during testing requires proper paperwork, precise labelling, and safe storage facilities.

Critical value detection and management in point-of-care testing is another crucial processing feature. A critical value is a diagnostic threshold at which medical intervention is mandatory to prevent death. In order to promote early detection and action, it is essential to define unambiguous and acceptable critical values. Notifying healthcare providers quickly and allowing for rapid response requires efficient communication systems, such as result verification, prioritization, and timely reporting.

Finally, processing isn't complete without the distribution of test results. Transmission of test results to authorized healthcare practitioners is what we call "result distribution." Timely decisions and clear lines of communication between the lab and healthcare teams rely on the distribution of results being both efficient and accurate. To aid in making educated clinical decisions and guarantee continuity of care, it is necessary to verify, interpret, priorities, and document results.

Centrifuging, aliquoting, properly managing, storing, transporting, and disposing of specimens, preserving the chain of custody, recognizing and handling important values, and disseminating results accurately and effectively all fall within the processing stage of laboratory testing. Laboratory results, patient care, and diagnostic quality can all benefit from a strict adherence to established protocols and best practices.

Chapter 11

Other Duties of a Phlebotomist

Phlebotomists' responsibilities extend beyond simply obtaining blood samples. Assisting in the collection of non-blood specimens like urine, farces, semen, and other sorts of samples is a common duty for them in addition to blood tests. These samples are crucial for medical research, patient monitoring, and diagnostic analysis. In addition to drawing blood, a phlebotomist may be responsible for collecting other types of specimens, such as urine, stool, and semen; supporting physicians with specimen collection; and handling and transporting these materials.

A phlebotomist's duties include giving patients detailed instructions for collecting urine. This is of utmost importance for urinalysis, drug testing, and other diagnostic uses involving the analysis of urine. The phlebotomist has the responsibility of informing the patient about the test's significance and directing them through the collection process. To reduce the possibility of contamination, patients should be instructed to wash their hands completely before collecting the urine sample. They should also be given a sterile container made for collecting urine and shown how to avoid touching the contents at any time. The patient should be instructed to urinate into the toilet as usual, then position the container midstream to capture a representative sample. The phlebotomist should then go through any extra documentation needs and stress the need of correctly labelling the specimen container with the patient's details, including name, date, and time of collection.

Phlebotomists may also be tasked with teaching patients how to collect farces for testing purposes. The collection of farces is required for faucal occult blood testing, stool culture, and parasite testing, among other diagnostic procedures. The phlebotomist's instructions for collecting stools should emphasize the use of a sterile, leak-proof container made for that purpose. In order to prevent contamination from urine and toilet paper, patients should be instructed to urinate before collecting the stool sample. They should be made aware of the importance of collecting a sample that is typical of the whole stool by taking a tiny amount from several different locations. Labelling the container correctly with the patient's details and keeping the appropriate records is also important.

Occasionally, phlebotomists will need to advise patients on how to collect semen. Collecting sperm is typically done for diagnostic purposes, ART treatments, and semen analysis. Patients requiring semen collection should be given a sterile, non-spermicidal container and instructed on how to use it properly, avoiding any contact with the contents. Masturbation, as well as the use of specific condoms or collection devices, should be among the collection procedures that patients are made aware of. In addition, they should be briefed on the need of confidentiality and a relaxed setting during the collection of the semen sample.

Phlebotomists may be asked to collect more than only blood, such as urine, faces, or semen. Swab samples might be anything from saliva to sputum to a tissue sample from the throat or nose. There could be different rules and requirements for various forms of collection. Phlebotomists should be well-versed in these protocols and give patients with precise directions to protect the safety and efficacy of the samples they draw.

When collecting specimens, phlebotomists frequently aid doctors and other medical staff. By working together, we can guarantee effective data collection. Following correct technique and aseptic principles, phlebotomists may help physicians collect and handle non-blood specimens, as well as assist with patient placement.

Phlebotomists are responsible for the safe collection, storage, and transportation of all specimens, not just blood. This includes using proper transport containers to keep specimens in pristine condition during transit, clearly labelling containers with patient information, and adhering to strict storage requirements. Phlebotomists are responsible for keeping track of specimens as they are transported and ensuring their safety until they reach the appropriate testing institution.

Phlebotomists are responsible for more than just collecting blood samples; they also instruct patients on how to properly collect urine, stool, and semen; assist physicians with specimen collection; and guarantee the safe handling and transport of all collected samples. These tasks are crucial to the success of diagnostic testing and patient care because they necessitate close attention to detail, open lines of contact with patients, and strict adherence to established protocols.

Patient Instructions for Urine Collection

Several diagnostic procedures necessitate collecting urine, the most frequent of which are urinalysis, culture, and sensitivity testing. Correct patient instructions are crucial for achieving consistent and precise outcomes. It is your duty as a phlebotomist to advise patients on how to collect urine in an understandable and thorough manner. Urine drug testing and general urine sample collection for diagnostic purposes will be the primary topics of this section, along with patient instructions for collecting urine.

Urine Drug Test

Patients require detailed instructions for taking urine drug testing in order to have reliable findings. Instructions for a urine drug test should cover the following topics:

Give an explanation for the test's point: To get started, you should inform the patient of the drug test's necessity and the reason a urine sample will be taken. Please specify any mandatory professional or legal criteria.

Instructions for getting ready for the test include telling the patient to fast for at least an hour before the procedure. Some drugs, vitamins, and herbal supplements may cause false positives or false negatives. It's vital to let the patient know that they should avoid these things unless absolutely necessary.

Timeframe for collection: Please be as detailed as possible regarding when a urine sample must be taken. This could be a random collection at some point during the day, or it could be the first void of the day. Make sure the patient is aware of the schedule and is able to stick to it.

Stress the significance of maintaining high standards of sanitation and hygiene in all aspects of sample collection. Before beginning the collection process, have the patient wash their hands well with soap and warm water. Reduce the potential for contamination by taking this measure.

Container for collecting urine: give the patient a clean, sterile container made for drug testing. Give instructions on how to prevent contamination by touching the inside of the container at any point. Show the patient how it's done if that's required.

To gather a representative sample, have the patient start peeing into the toilet and then place the collecting container midstream. The beginning and end of the urine stream are less likely to be contaminated using this procedure.

Inform the patient of the amount of urine that will be needed for the test. A minimal volume of 30 mL (1 oz.) is usually adequate. Make sure the patient knows how much you need and have them collect enough.

The specimen container must be clearly labelled with the patient's name, the date and time of collection, and any other pertinent information. Inform the patient that they must include a completed form with their urine sample.

Instructions on how to properly preserve and transport the urine sample should be provided. The sample must be properly packaged and delivered to the appropriate staff or laboratory as soon as possible. Specify any necessary storage conditions, such as temperature and humidity.

Patient Instructions for Stool Collection

The collection of farces is required for faucal occult blood testing, stool culture, and parasite testing, among other diagnostic procedures. Correct patient instructions are essential for reliable outcomes. Instructing a patient to take a stool sample should emphasize the following points:

Give an explanation for the test's point: To begin, you should talk to the patient about why you need a stool sample. Explain how this test will aid in the patient's diagnosis and treatment.

Instruct the patient to abstain from any substances, including food, medication, and supplements, that may affect the findings of the test. Stool cultures can be impacted by medications like antibiotics and antacids. Give a detailed list of substances that should be avoided, and outline why it's crucial that they be avoided.

Container for collection: Give the patient a sterile, airtight container made for holding farces. Give instructions on how to prevent contamination by touching the inside of the container at any point. If you want reliable results from your tests, you must use the container given, not something from about the house.

Put an emphasis on maintaining high standards of cleanliness before, during, and after the collection process. Tell the patient to use soap and warm water to fully cleanse their hands before you begin collecting. To prevent contamination, you should also use disposable toilet paper and keep the toilet seat clean.

Collecting the sample: Tell us when you'd like the stool sample to be taken. The collection of many samples over the course of several days may be necessary in some situations. Make sure the patient is aware of the schedule and is able to stick to it.

Method of Collection: Have the Patient Collect Samples of Stool from Several Locations in the Bowel Movement. This guarantees a fair sampling for scientific analysis. It's crucial that the sample doesn't get ruined by things like urine or too much toilet paper.

Sample size: let the patient know how much stool is needed for the analysis. The typical sample size is around the size of a walnut, or about two to three tablespoons. Make sure the patient knows how much you need and have them collect enough.

The specimen container must be clearly labelled with the patient's name, the date and time of collection, and any other pertinent information. Instruct the patient to fill out any paperwork or forms that must be sent along with the stool sample.

Storage and transportation: Specify how long the stool sample can be kept at room temperature and how it should be transported. A biohazard bag or other airtight container should be used to store the sample. Specify any necessary storage conditions, such as temperature and humidity.

Patient Instructions for Semen Collection

Collecting sperm is typically done for fertility testing, IVF, and other assisted reproductive techniques. Accurate results and patient comfort and privacy depend on doctors giving patients clear and sensitive instructions. Helping patients understand why and how semen is collected is an important part of becoming a phlebotomist. Instructions for obtaining sperm from patients should emphasize the following points:

Defend the necessity of the collection by explaining: Before collecting any sperm, it's important to talk to the patient about why you're doing it and how it will help with their diagnosis or therapy. Talk about the analytical methods that will be used on the sample.

Tell the patient how long they need to abstain from sexual activity before you can collect their sperm. For 2–5 days ahead to the collection, patients are often asked to refrain from all sexual activity. Make sure the patient knows how crucial it is to follow these directions for the best possible outcome.

Patients may be instructed to collect the semen sample by masturbation, a specialized condom, or a collection device, depending on the individual requirements. Provide detailed explanations of each approach and any supporting documents that may be needed for the approach that wins.

Stress the significance of discretion and ease of movement during semen collecting. The best environment for a patient is one in which they feel at ease and can give their whole attention to the task at hand. Insist that they make the space calm and undisrupted.

Give the patient a container made for collecting sperm that is sterile and does not contain spermicidal agents. Tell the patient to keep their hands off the contents of the container at all times. If it's required, show them how it's done.

Collection Timeframe It is important to specify when the semen sample to be collected. The patient may need to collect the sample immediately after ejaculation, or within a certain time limit, depending on the individual criteria. Make sure the patient is aware of the schedule and is able to stick to it.

The amount of semen needed for the test or procedure should be communicated to the patient. A volume between 1 and 5 milliliters is usually adequate. Make sure the patient knows how much you need and that they collect enough.

The specimen container must be clearly labelled with the patient's name, the date and time of collection, and any other pertinent information. Please have the patient fill out any paperwork or forms that will be sent with the semen sample.

Non-Blood Specimen Collections

Phlebotomists may be asked to collect more than only blood, such as urine, feces, or semen. Swab samples might be anything from saliva to sputum to a tissue sample from the throat or nose. There could be different rules and requirements for various forms of collection. Instructions for collecting specimens other than blood should generally follow these guidelines:

Defend the necessity of the collection by explaining: Explain to the patient how the specimen will help in making a diagnosis or determining a course of treatment. Specify the analyses or other treatments that will be applied to the sample.

Tell the patient what they need to do to get ready for you to take their specimens. In order to collect saliva or throat swabs, for instance, the patient may need to fast for a certain amount of time.

Instructions on how to capture this species in particular should be given in great detail. Saliva samples can be collected by spitting into a container, sputum samples can be collected by coughing hard, and swab samples can be collected from a wound, the throat, or the nose. If it is required, show a demonstration of the method.

Offer the patient a sterile collection vessel that is designed to hold their particular specimen. Describe what to do to prevent sample contamination when handling the container and how to pack it safely for shipment.

Collection Timeframe Indicate when you'd like the specimen to be collected. Early morning collection is recommended for some items, such as sputum. Make sure the patient is aware of the schedule and is able to stick to it.

How many samples were taken: Make sure the patient knows how much of a specimen is needed for the surgery. Specify in detail the minimum and maximum amounts they should collect in order to obtain representative data.

Labelling and documentation: Make sure the patient's information and the correct paperwork or papers are clearly labelled on the specimen container.

Give directions on how to keep the specimen safe and how to transfer it. The specimen must be delivered to the laboratory or testing facility within a certain time frame and temperature range.

Assisting Physicians with Specimen Collection

Helping doctors collect specimens from patients is a crucial part of your job as a phlebotomist. Tasks may include assisting the doctor during procedures or collecting, transporting, and processing specimens. In this article, we'll go through all the ways in which you can help doctors out during the specimen collection process.

If you want to help doctors gather specimens, you need to know what they need for each surgery. Knowing what kind of specimen is required, how to collect it, and if any additional care must be taken is all part of this. Get all of your questions answered and make sure you understand the doctor's expectations by talking to them before the surgery.

You will have to make sure the collection area is clean and sterile before the procedure begins. Preparation entails accumulating and setting up things like specimen collection containers, swabs, and other similar items. Make sure everything the doctor needs is organized, sterilized, and within easy reach.

You'll be relied on heavily to aid the doctor in specimen collection processes. Helping a patient may require holding instruments or equipment, guiding them through a series of steps, or repositioning them. To aid ensure patient comfort and cooperation, it is crucial to rigorously adhere to the physician's recommendations and have a calm and comforting demeanor.

You will be in charge of taking care of and labeling specimen containers after collection. This includes checking the seals to make sure no leakage or contamination has occurred. Proper identification and monitoring of specimens throughout the testing process rely on labels that are both accurate and legible. Make sure the patient's information on the label coincides with that on the paperwork.

You'll have to take care of specimen storage and transport after you bring them in. Depending on the type of specimen, special care must be taken during storage. Transport and storage must be handled according to the doctor's orders or the laboratory's protocols. Also, make sure the specimens are well-protected from damage and leaking in their packaging before sending them off.

Strict infection control procedures must be upheld at all times when helping doctors gather specimens. This includes washing one's hands before and after handling specimens, wearing gloves, masks, and gowns as necessary, and following sterile procedures. To prevent the spread of disease, it is imperative that proper precautions be taken and infection control measures implemented at all times.

Accurate documentation is essential when helping doctors collect specimens. Maintain complete and well-organized records of all samples taken, including patient data, collection details, and notes. Notify the doctor or lab staff of any concerns or irregularities as soon as possible, and make sure all the required paperwork is included with the specimens for efficient tracking and analysis.

Handling and Transporting Non-Blood Specimen

As a phlebotomist, you may be tasked with more than just aiding doctors with specimen collection; you may also have to handle and transport non-blood specimens to the lab. Urine, farces, sputum, and other body fluids are all considered specimens. Preserving specimen integrity and guaranteeing reliable laboratory testing relies on careful handling and transportation. Important things to remember when transporting and managing specimens that aren't blood:

It is crucial to use containers made for the particular type of specimen being collected while working with non-blood specimens. Urine, stool, and sputum samples, among others, need to be collected in containers that will keep their contents safe from contamination. Seal all containers securely and clearly label them with the patient's name and other pertinent information.

Certain conditions must be met before transporting non-blood specimens to ensure their stability and integrity. It may be necessary to refrigerate certain samples, maintain others at ambient temperature, or shield others from light. Learn the precise requirements for storing each type of specimen until shipment, and do it responsibly.

Urine and microbiological samples, for example, may need to be kept at a specific temperature throughout shipment. To keep things within the desired temperature range, use insulated containers or the proper coolants, like ice packs or refrigerants. Protect and insulate samples so that they don't experience temperature changes that could compromise their quality.

It is possible that infectious pathogens could be present in some non-blood specimens, making them a biohazard. To properly handle and transport biohazardous specimens, you should take the appropriate safeguards, as outlined in standard operating procedures and as supplemented by your healthcare facility. Wear protective gear like gloves and aprons when handling specimens, and make sure the containers are airtight to avoid contamination.

When shipping specimens other than blood, it is essential that they be properly documented and labelled. Mark each specimen container with the patient's name, the date it was collected, and any identifying numbers. Make sure the specimens are safely attached to any necessary paperwork, including requisition forms or laboratory request forms.

Timely transit to the laboratory is essential for the preservation of non-blood specimens. Make that samples are delivered on time and according to the established transport plan. If transport delays are anticipated, such as overnight storage, the specimen must be properly stored to ensure its viability during the waiting period.

Keep the lab staff in the loop on how non-blood specimens should be handled and transported. If there are any unique circumstances or concerns, such as a pressing need for expedited processing or rigorous testing standards, please let them know right away. If the laboratory has supplied special instructions for shipping procedures or additional paperwork, be sure to adhere to those as well.

Laboratory testing relies on the accuracy of the specimens collected, and phlebotomists play a crucial part in this by guaranteeing the integrity of non-blood specimens during handling and transport. Important parts of this procedure include being compliant, taking precautions against infection, and documenting everything thoroughly.

Chapter 12

Core Knowledge

The fundamentals of phlebotomy practice are the focus here. Blood samples are collected from patients for use in diagnostics and transfusions, making phlebotomy technicians an integral part of the healthcare team. To do their jobs effectively and securely, they need in-depth knowledge of a wide range of subjects.

Phlebotomy technicians are essential to the healthcare system since they are responsible for obtaining blood samples for further examination in the lab. Patient identification must be confirmed, the method must be explained to the patient, an acceptable venipuncture site must be chosen, the venipuncture procedure must be performed, and blood samples must be properly labelled and stored. Possible additional duties include handling and transporting specimens.

Phlebotomy technicians need to know a wide range of medical terminology. Knowing the lingo associated with anatomy, physiology, laboratory tests, and clinical procedures is essential. In order to effectively communicate with other medical professionals and to properly document patient information, knowledge of medical language is crucial.

When doing phlebotomy, it is essential to utilize aseptic technique to avoid contaminating the blood or other potentially vulnerable parts of the body with bacteria or other pathogens. In order to prevent the spread of disease, phlebotomy technicians must work in a clean, sterile atmosphere and always wear the necessary protective gear.

Phlebotomists should know how various blood components work and what they are made of. A thorough understanding of the components of blood is required, including RBCs, WBCs, platelets, plasma, and more. Technicians in the field of phlebotomy benefit from an understanding of blood components since it allows them to perform their jobs more effectively.

Phlebotomy technicians must be familiar with blood group systems such the ABO and Rh. Transfusing incompatible blood can cause life-threatening reactions due to the presence of antigens on the surface of the red blood cells that are unique to each blood group. Technicians in the field of phlebotomy are responsible for collecting and labelling blood samples for transfusions, which requires them to correctly identify blood types and guarantee compatibility.

Phlebotomy technicians rely on their knowledge of vascular anatomy to locate healthy veins for venipuncture. Successful blood draws require an understanding of the human venous system and its placement. Complications can be kept to a minimum and patient comfort can be maintained with an understanding of vascular architecture.

Technicians in the field of phlebotomy should have a foundational knowledge of the cardiovascular system. Knowing this helps them assess patient circumstances and react correctly during venipuncture operations, as well as understand the significance of their role in collecting blood samples.

Hemostasis and coagulation, the body's capacity to stop bleeding and create blood clots, are concepts that phlebotomy technicians should be familiar with. Phlebotomists who are well-versed in the mechanisms of hemostasis are better equipped to deal with complications including excessive bleeding and clotting disorders that may emerge during or after venipuncture.

Mistakes that occur before to laboratory testing are known as pre-analytical errors and include things like erroneous patient identification, incorrect specimen collection or handling, and inadequate labelling. Because of the serious consequences they can have on the precision and dependability of laboratory test results, phlebotomy technicians must be aware of and take measures to prevent these mistakes.

United States federal law protecting healthcare workers from needlestick injuries and bloodborne diseases is called the Needlestick Safety and Prevention Act. In order to guarantee their own and others' safety in the healthcare setting, phlebotomy technicians should be familiar with this legislation and follow its requirements.

A phlebotomy technician's duties include keeping detailed records and submitting timely reports. They must document pertinent patient data, venipuncture technique specifics, and any occurrences or difficulties that arise. An accurate medical record can only be maintained by meticulous documentation, which also improves communication between doctors.

Phlebotomy technicians should be able to communicate well both verbally and nonverbally. They frequently communicate with patients, answering questions, addressing concerns, and outlining upcoming operations. Building rapport, making sure patients are comfortable, and providing excellent treatment all come down to good communication.

Professionalism and ethical conduct are two of the most important qualities of a phlebotomy technician. They have a responsibility to protect patients' privacy, treat them with dignity, act ethically, and put their well-being first. Maintaining a professional demeanor benefits both patients and the phlebotomy field as a whole.

Knowledge of aseptic technique, blood components, blood group systems, vascular anatomy, cardiovascular system, hemostasis and coagulation, pre-analytical errors, needlestick safety, documenting and reporting, communication skills, professionalism, and ethical standards are all essential for phlebotomy technicians.

Phlebotomy technicians improve the quality of patient care and laboratory testing when they have the foundational knowledge necessary to do their jobs correctly, safely, and professionally.

Role of Phlebotomy Technicians

Technicians trained in phlebotomy are essential in the healthcare industry because of the importance of their work in collecting and processing blood samples for use in diagnosis and transfusions. The collection of blood samples from patients is their number one priority. Phlebotomy technicians need technical expertise, medical knowledge, and people skills to carry out their duties. In this article, we will delve into the phlebotomy technician's job description.

Patient identification is an essential part of a phlebotomy technician's job. Patients' identities are checked before every venipuncture is performed to make that the right person is getting the right tests or treatment. This is done by confirming the patient's identity by verifying the information on the requisition form or electronic order with the patient's identification bracelet, name, and date of birth.

After verifying the patient's identity, phlebotomy technicians talk to them. They make sure the patient is prepared for the blood draw by thoroughly explaining the process to them. In order to allay the patient's concerns and secure their permission for the operation, clear and concise communication is crucial. Technicians performing phlebotomy must also reassure patients by addressing their fears and reassuring them during the operation.

The phlebotomy technician is also responsible for picking out good venipuncture sites. They need to locate open, easily reached veins from which to draw blood. Venipuncture is typically performed in the antecubital fossa (inner elbow), the dorsum of the hand, or the forearm. Factors such as the patient's age, medical condition, and the intended tests may influence the decision about the testing location.

Phlebotomy workers need to be proficient in the venipuncture operation itself. Blood is drawn from the chosen vein using sterile needles and collection tubes. To successfully draw blood, the needle must be inserted into the vein at the correct angle and depth, and the needle must be withdrawn using the same methodical approach. Technicians in the field of phlebotomy must be comfortable working with patients of all ages, from children to the elderly.

Phlebotomists are responsible for the safe and secure labelling and storage of blood samples after they have been collected. The sample's integrity and traceability depend on its proper labelling. Patients' names, the time and date of collection, and any other pertinent information must be clearly labelled on each tube. It is equally important to properly store and transport specimens to the laboratory to preserve the quality of the samples and guarantee reliable test findings.

Technicians in phlebotomy may also be responsible for handling and transporting specimens. Separating the serum or plasma from the cellular components of a blood sample requires centrifugation, and if necessary, aliquoting the sample into smaller tubes and meticulously recording the specimens for laboratory testing. distinct types of specimens require distinct procedures to guarantee safe transport and arrival at the lab.

Terminology

Phlebotomists rely heavily on their knowledge of and facility with medical terminology for two reasons: communicating with other medical staff and accurately documenting patient information. Phlebotomy technicians must be conversant with a wide range of medical jargon because they are used frequently in their everyday work. Let's take a look at a few phlebotomy buzzwords:

Puncturing a vein with a needle for the purpose of drawing blood, either for testing or treatment, is known as venipuncture. Phlebotomy technicians typically obtain blood samples by venipuncture.

The antecubital fossa is a vein-rich area on the inner aspect of the elbow. Because of its convenient location and large, easily accessible veins, the antecubital fossa is frequently employed as a blood collection site.

Hematology refers to the study of blood and blood problems within the medical field. To enable reliable testing and analysis of blood samples, phlebotomy technicians frequently interact with hematologists and other laboratory personnel.

Serum is the yellowish-clear fluid that is collected after blood has been clotted and the blood cells and clotting factors have been removed. Phlebotomists are responsible for collecting and properly processing serum samples, which are used in a wide variety of laboratory procedures.

Plasma is the remaining liquid after blood cells and clotting components have been removed. Proteins, hormones, electrolytes, and waste products are just some of what you'll find in plasma. Plasma samples may be collected by phlebotomists for use in diagnostic procedures or in the manufacture of blood products like plasma-derived treatments.

Hemoglobin is the oxygen-carrying protein molecule in red blood cells. It also transports carbon dioxide from the tissues back to the lungs. Blood samples are often analyzed for hemoglobin levels in order to diagnose anemia and evaluate the body's ability to transport oxygen.

Hemolysis refers to the release of hemoglobin into the surrounding fluid or serum after red blood cells have been damaged or destroyed. Certain blood tests can be impacted by hemolysis because it can impede the measurement of specific analytes.

Coagulation refers to the creation of a blood clot, which aids in the prevention of excessive bleeding. Technicians in the field of phlebotomy need to understand how blood clotting works and how it affects the collection and processing of blood samples.

An anticoagulant is a drug that slows or stops the coagulation of blood. When collecting blood for testing, anticoagulants are sometimes added to the tubes to prevent the sample from clotting. Phlebotomists have the responsibility of ensuring that the correct anticoagulant is mixed with each blood sample.

The condition known as thrombosis occurs when a blood clot, sometimes called a thrombus, forms inside a blood vessel and blocks blood flow. Technicians performing venipuncture should be familiar with the causes of thrombosis and how to prevent the formation of blood clots.

Phlebitis is vein inflammation brought on by infection or venipuncture-related discomfort. The symptoms of phlebitis include tenderness, redness, and swelling near the affected vein. Technicians doing phlebotomy should be especially watchful for symptoms of phlebitis at the venipuncture site.

Hemoconcentration occurs when the tourniquet is applied to a vein for an extended period of time, increasing the concentration of cells and substances in the blood. Hemoconcentration can cause falsely elevated analyte concentrations, which can throw off the results of a blood test.

A specimen's "Chain of Custody" is a record of every step taken with it from the moment it was collected to the moment it was tested. Forensic and legal applications absolutely require a secure and verifiable chain of custody to guarantee the authenticity and provenance of a specimen.

Phlebotomy technicians can better serve their patients, other medical professionals, and the healthcare system as a whole if they have a firm grasp of medical terminologies like these and others. It also ensures the quality and reliability of laboratory test results and promotes efficient collaboration.

Aseptic Technique

When doing phlebotomy, it is essential to utilize aseptic technique to avoid contaminating the blood or other potentially vulnerable parts of the body with bacteria or other pathogens. In order to keep patients safe and reduce the likelihood of infection, it is essential to keep the facility clean and sterile at all times. Let's take a closer look at what makes phlebotomy aseptic as possible.

Hand Hygiene: Phlebotomy technicians should always wash their hands before and after handling a patient. This requires either using an alcohol-based hand sanitizer or washing one's hands with soap and water for at least 20 seconds. Cross-contamination can be prevented, and transient bacteria eliminated by practicing good hand hygiene.

Phlebotomy technicians should take precautions against exposure to bloodborne pathogens and other infectious materials by wearing protective gear such as gloves, masks, and goggles. Gloves must be worn at all times when interacting with patients and thrown away after usage. Wearing a mask and goggles can protect you from inhaled particulates and splashed bodily fluids.

Aseptic conditions require regular and thorough disinfection of all surfaces and tools. Technicians in the field of phlebotomy should use the proper disinfectants while cleaning and sanitizing items like phlebotomy carts and work surfaces. This aids in the reduction or elimination of environmental microorganisms.

Phlebotomists are responsible for ensuring that all needles, collection tubes, and blood culture flasks used during venipuncture are sterile and have not been contaminated. The collecting location should be kept clean by using sterile gloves during the operation.

Phlebotomy technicians are required to disinfect the skin with an antiseptic solution before performing venipuncture. Commonly used antiseptics include chlorhexidine and povidone-iodine. This decreases the amount of bacteria on the skin and the likelihood of bringing diseases into the body.

Phlebotomy technicians should not contact the venipuncture site or the interior of collection tubes with their bare hands or gloves at any time throughout the venipuncture procedure to prevent the spread of infection. The integrity of a blood sample or the introduction of microbes into the bloodstream can be compromised by touch contamination.

After a venipuncture operation is complete, the needle and any other sharps should be disposed of in a puncture-resistant container. This assures the proper disposal of contaminated sharps and reduces the risk of needlestick injuries.

Environmental controls involve ensuring that phlebotomy technicians work in a sanitary environment devoid of debris and other potential health hazards. Contamination in the air can be reduced with good ventilation and airflow.

Phlebotomists and other medical staff are also protected from potential infection when aseptic procedures are followed during the blood collection process. Phlebotomy technicians help make healthcare facilities safer and more conducive to providing high-quality service to patients by adhering to these standards.

Blood Components

Blood is a crucial bodily fluid that helps with things like oxygen transportation, immune system support, and temperature maintenance. Several parts make up the whole, and they all serve distinct purposes. Phlebotomy technicians' knowledge of blood types and components is essential to their success on the job. Let's take a look at what makes blood what it is:

Erythrocytes, often known as red blood cells (RBCs), are the most common type of blood cell and are essential for life because they carry oxygen from the lungs to the rest of the body. They have a protein called hemoglobin in them that carries oxygen across the body and attaches to molecules of oxygen. Carbon dioxide is a byproduct of cellular metabolism, and RBCs help remove it from the tissues and return it to the lungs to be exhaled.

White blood cells, also called leukocytes, are an important part of the immune system that helps the body fight off infections and other disorders. Antigen-detecting and -destroying cells, antibody production, and immune response regulation all fall under their purview. Neutrophils, lymphocytes, monocytes, eosinophils, and basophils are all forms of WBCs that serve diverse purposes in the immune system.

Platelets, also known as thrombocytes, are fragments of larger cells that are essential to hemostasis. Platelets clump together to create a clog at the site of a blood vessel injury. They also secrete clotting factors, which set in motion the chain of events that results in a solid clot of blood.

Plasma is the liquid portion of blood, constituting around 55 percent of the total volume. It consists of a wide variety of chemicals, including water, proteins, electrolytes, hormones, minerals, waste products, and more. Plasma helps keep the body's fluid levels and pH stable, and it also carries nutrients, hormones, and waste products. Antibodies and other immune system proteins are also present.

Blood Group Systems

Human blood is categorized into different blood groups based on whether or not certain antigens are present on the surface of the red blood cells. Blood type is determined by these antigens, which has important consequences for things like organ transplants and blood transfusions. The ABO system and the Rh system are the two most common types of blood groups. Let's have a look at the significance of these structures:

The ABO blood group system classifies blood into four primary types—A, B, AB, and O—based on whether or not the red blood cells carry A and B antigens. People with blood type A have A antigens, those with blood type B have B antigens, those with blood type AB have both A and B antigens, and those with blood type O do not. Furthermore, the presence of antibodies (anti-A and anti-B) in the plasma is used by the ABO system to categorize blood types. Mismatched blood types can cause life-threatening transfusion reactions, making knowledge of the ABO blood group system essential for safe blood transfusions.

The Rh system classifies blood as either Rh-positive (Rh+) or Rh-negative (Rh-) depending on whether or not the red blood cells carry the Rh antigen (also called the D antigen). People who are Rh+ have the Rh antigen, while those who are Rh- do not. Rh incompatibility between a Rh- mother and a Rh+ fetus can result in hemolytic illness of the infant, making the Rh system especially important in cases of pregnancy. Blood transfusions must be Rh compatible to avoid giving Rh-people an immune response.

Other than the ABO and Rh systems, which share antigenic markers, there are several more, including the Kell, Duffy, Kidd, and Lewis systems. The clinical relevance of these systems varies, and they may only be of use in very narrow cases, such as those involving organ transplant incompatibilities or extremely rare blood illnesses.

Vascular Anatomy

The term "vascular anatomy" is used to describe the study of the circulatory system's blood vessels. Phlebotomy technicians must be well-versed in vascular anatomy in order to successfully locate and access veins for blood collection. Successful venipuncture procedures and minimal complications can be ensured by familiarity with the anatomy and physiology of blood arteries. Now we'll take a look at the fundamentals of vascular anatomy:

Blood vessels called arteries convey oxygen-rich blood away from the heart to be distributed to the body's tissues and organs. In order to endure the intense pressure created by the heart's constant beating, arteries have strong, thick walls. The capillaries are the tiniest blood vessels and are formed when arteries divide into arterioles.

Capillaries are very small capillaries with very thin walls that link arteries to veins. They play a crucial role in the transfer of oxygen and nutrients from the circulatory system to the body's cells. The extensive network of capillaries throughout the body facilitates the effective transport of oxygen, carbon dioxide, nutrients, and waste items between the blood and the cells.

Veins are blood arteries responsible for returning oxygen-poor blood from the body's tissues to the heart. Veins, in contrast to arteries, have more permeable walls and are equipped with valves that keep blood from reversing direction. The superior and inferior vena cava are the two biggest veins, carrying blood back to the right atrium of the heart.

Superficial veins, deep veins, and perforator veins are all components of the venous system. Superficial veins are those closest to the skin's surface, and they are the ones most commonly accessed during venipuncture. It's common for arteries to work in tandem with the deeper, more internal veins. The perforator veins are the conduits between the superficial and deep veins; they are valved to prevent backflow.

Technicians in the field of phlebotomy need an in-depth knowledge of the circulatory system in order to choose safe venipuncture sites that provide the least amount of pain and risk to patients. They must locate veins by sight and touch, evaluate vein size and health, and modify their approach according to the patient's age and medical history.

Cardiovascular System

Blood, oxygen, nutrition, hormones, and waste products are all transported throughout the body through the cardiovascular system, also known as the circulatory system. It's essential for homeostasis and the proper functioning of numerous bodily systems and tissues. Phlebotomy technicians must have a thorough knowledge of the circulatory system in order to perform venipuncture and properly manage blood samples. Let's take a closer look at the cardiovascular system and its primary parts and functions:

The heart is a muscular organ situated somewhat to the left of the center of the chest. It pumps blood through the circulatory system by repeatedly contracting and relaxing like a muscle. The atria (singular: atrium) and ventricles (plural: ventricles) are the upper and lower chambers of the heart, respectively. The ventricles pump blood out to the body, whereas the atria take in blood that has been pumped there from the body.

The vessels of the circulatory system carry blood to all parts of the body. The human circulatory system consists of arteries, veins, and capillaries. Arteries are blood vessels that transport oxygenated blood from the heart to the rest of the body. Blood that has been oxygenated in the tissues is carried back to the heart via veins. Capillaries are the thin-walled, small blood vessels that link arteries to veins and facilitate the transport of oxygen, nutrients, and waste products from the blood to the tissues they serve.

In the cardiovascular system, blood flows as a specialized fluid. The many parts of blood are the erythrocytes (red blood cells), leukocytes (white blood cells), platelets (thrombocytes), and plasma. Plasma is the liquid component that transports nutrients, hormones, and waste materials, while red blood cells bring oxygen to the tissues, white blood cells play a part in the immune response, and platelets are engaged in blood clotting.

What we mean when we talk about "blood pressure" is the pressure that the blood is putting on the artery and capillary walls. Systolic pressure (when the heart is actively contracting) and diastolic pressure (when the heart is at rest) are the two numbers used to determine this. Sufficient blood flow to the organs and tissues relies on a healthy blood pressure level. High or low blood pressure levels may signal heart disease.

The term "circulation" is used to describe how the heart pumps blood throughout the body. Systemic circulation and pulmonary circulation are the two most common forms. The pulmonary circulatory system transports deoxygenated blood from the heart to the lungs for oxygenation and returns oxygenated blood to the heart, whereas the systemic circulatory system delivers oxygenated blood to the body's tissues and organs.

Hemostasis and Coagulation

When a blood vessel is damaged, the body immediately begins the physiological process of hemostasis, which stops the bleeding. There is a complex set of systems at work to keep blood fluid under normal conditions and to clot it when a blood artery is injured to prevent excessive bleeding. Phlebotomy technicians, who handle blood samples for testing, must have a thorough understanding of hemostasis and coagulation. Let's have a look at what makes hemostasis and coagulation tick:

Vasoconstriction:

The narrowing of blood vessels in response to injury, which helps to control bleeding. Smooth muscle contraction in the walls of blood vessels is the primary mediator of vasoconstriction.

Platelets are fragments of larger cells that circulate in the blood and play a crucial role in clotting and other forms of hemostasis. Platelets are activated when they stick to the site of a blood vessel injury. Platelets clump together after activation to create a temporary plug that aids in bleeding control.

Blood clots are the result of a complicated set of enzyme processes known as the coagulation cascade. There are many different proteins, enzymes, and clotting factors involved. Blood vessel injury initiates the intrinsic process, while tissue injury sets off the extrinsic pathway.

Fibrin Formation:

The transformation of soluble fibrinogen into insoluble fibrin strands is the final stage of the coagulation cascade. Fibrin creates a mesh-like network that supports the platelet plug and helps the blood clot to stick together.

After a clot forms, a process known as retraction takes place, during which the platelets contract and the fibrin strands rearrange themselves. The clot's strength is increased, and the injured region is diminished as a result of retraction.

Once the damaged blood vessel has healed, a process called fibrinolysis begins to break down and destroy the clot. Plasmin is an enzyme that breaks down fibrin strands and dissolves the clot so that blood flow can resume normally.

Pre-Analytical Errors

Errors that occur before a blood sample is tested or analyzed are called pre-analytical errors. Incorrect diagnoses, unwarranted therapies, and substandard care for patients are all possible outcomes of such mistakes in the laboratory. By adhering to standard procedures and best practices, phlebotomy technicians play a crucial role in reducing the contamination of samples before analysis. Let's talk about some frequent pre-analytical mistakes and how to avoid them:

Mislabeled or misplaced blood samples are examples of patient identification errors that can lead to false positives. Phlebotomists can avoid making these mistakes by double-checking the patient's identity with two identifiers a name and a date of birth or a unique ID number before drawing blood. At each stage, from collecting samples to labeling and transporting them, verifying the patient's identity is crucial.

The integrity and quality of a blood sample can be jeopardized by human error that occurs during the collection process. Technicians in the field of phlebotomy are responsible for ensuring that patients are properly prepared for venipuncture or fingerstick procedures, including fasting if necessary. They need to collect the right amount of blood for each test using sterile equipment like needles and tubes. If numerous tests are needed, it is also important to collect samples in the precise order to prevent contamination.

Errors in Specimen Handling and Transport Hemolysis (the destruction of red blood cells), contamination, or specimen degradation can occur if blood samples are handled improperly or transported for too long. Blood samples should be handled carefully by phlebotomists, who should label, seal, and store them at the correct temperature. They need to use appropriate containers and get the samples to the lab on time, per predetermined procedures.

Mistakes in Documentation:

In the pre-analytical phase, good documentation is crucial for tracing and following blood samples. Technicians doing phlebotomy should keep meticulous records of all patient interactions and data, including patient identification, collection date and time, test orders, and any pertinent instructions or observations. Errors in sample identification, processing, and reporting of results can be avoided with thorough documentation.

Misunderstandings:

Correct specimen collection and management rely on clear understanding between phlebotomy workers, patients, and other medical staff. Phlebotomy technicians are responsible for effectively communicating with patients about the collection process, including pre- and post-collection care. They should also talk to the lab techs and let them know if there is anything they need to know before doing testing.

Needlestick Safety and Prevention Act

The Needlestick Safety and Prevention Act (NSPA) is a landmark federal law passed in 2000 with the goal of reducing the risk of needlestick injuries and other forms of bloodborne pathogen exposure among healthcare workers in the workplace. This law is vital in preventing the spread of blood-borne infections including HIV, hepatitis B, and hepatitis C among healthcare workers by reducing the likelihood of needlestick injuries. The NSPA requires healthcare facilities to educate and train their staff on how to prevent needlestick injuries.

The NSPA mandates the use of less dangerous medical equipment in healthcare facilities. The danger of needlestick injuries can be reduced with the use of equipment like needleless systems and sharps with engineered sharps injury protection (SESIP). Needlestick injuries can be greatly reduced and healthcare workers' safety improved if healthcare facilities adopt these safer medical devices.

The NSPA stresses the importance of healthcare facilities developing and implementing an Exposure Control Plan (ECP), in addition to the use of safer medical devices. The Exposure Control Plan (ECP) is an all-encompassing strategy with the goal of reducing the likelihood of occupational exposure to bloodborne pathogens. Risk assessments, engineering controls, work practice controls, the provision of personal protective equipment (PPE), immunization programmers, and reporting and follow-up processes for needlestick injuries are all part of this system. The best way for healthcare facilities to protect their staff from harm is to implement an ECP that emphasizes eliminating the potential for needlesticks and other sources of bloodborne pathogen exposure in the workplace.

Documenting and Reporting

Documentation and reporting in the medical field must be accurate and comprehensive. Keeping accurate records and filing reports is essential in the field of phlebotomy since it helps with patient safety, legal compliance, and the smooth flow of information between healthcare practitioners.

Maintaining a paper trail is essential for providing uninterrupted service to patients. Documentation allows doctors to keep track of a patient's whole medical history, from lab results to diagnosis to treatments to drugs. This data helps doctors determine the best course of therapy for their patients, monitor their progress, and identify any problems early on. As an added bonus, thorough documentation encourages interdisciplinary collaboration, which helps doctors from various backgrounds work together to give patients the best care possible.

There are legal and regulatory requirements for recording and reporting information. Having a complete record of the care that was delivered to the patient is essential for legal and liability reasons. Documentation can serve as proof to support the activities done by healthcare practitioners and assure compliance with legal and regulatory standards in the event of a legal dispute or malpractice claim. In addition, quality improvement activities and patient safety depend on accurate reporting of accidents, errors, and other problems. Healthcare providers can increase patient safety and the quality of care overall by focusing on prevention after recognizing problem areas.

Importance of Verbal and Nonverbal Communication

Clear and accurate information exchange, building relationships with patients, and fostering patient-centered care all depend on effective verbal and nonverbal communication between healthcare providers and their patients.

Words and language are used to train patients, share information, and have therapeutic talks with them through verbal communication. Phlebotomy technicians must be able to explain procedures, acquire informed consent, and answer any concerns or issues patients may have through clear and simple verbal communication. Phlebotomy technicians can increase patient compliance and decrease anxiety or dread during blood collection procedures by speaking clearly, avoiding medical jargon, and actively listening to their patients.

Tone of voice, facial expressions, and body language are all examples of nonverbal communication. Emotions, attitudes, and intentions can frequently be communicated more effectively through these nonverbal indicators than through words alone. Phlebotomy relies heavily on nonverbal cues to provide a relaxing and reassuring space for patients. Phlebotomy technicians can improve their patients' experiences by keeping a soothing demeanor, employing suitable body language, and listening attentively to their concerns.

In addition, phlebotomy technicians can evaluate their patients' levels of pain, distress, and discomfort through the use of nonverbal cues. To maximize patient comfort and safety, phlebotomy technicians should pay close attention to nonverbal indications such as facial expressions, body language, and changes in vital signs.

Professionalism & Ethical Standards

The phlebotomy profession places a premium on professionalism and ethical behavior. Technicians in the field of phlebotomy are held to a very high standard of professionalism and ethics in order to guarantee the health and well-being of their patients. Let's have a look at what makes a phlebotomist professional and ethical:

Phlebotomy technicians need to be knowledgeable, skilled, and able to do their jobs in a safe and effective manner. Phlebotomists need to keep up with the latest developments in the field by attending continuing education classes and workshops. Competence demonstration is essential for producing trustworthy test results and protecting patients.

Phlebotomy technicians deal with confidential patient information such as medical history and lab findings. To protect patient privacy and meet legal and ethical obligations, they must adhere to stringent confidentiality and privacy standards. Building trust and promoting a secure healthcare environment are two outcomes of protecting patients' privacy and keeping their information confidential.

Displaying proper demeanor, outlook, and social skills are hallmarks of a phlebotomist's professionalism. When engaging with patients, coworkers, and other healthcare professionals, phlebotomy technicians should show respect, empathy, and cultural awareness. They should always look presentable, speak clearly, and work well with others as part of a larger healthcare team.

Ethical Decisions and Judgements Phlebotomy technologists make are informed by ethical norms. Autonomy, beneficence, nonmaleficence, and justice are all ethical ideals that they should uphold. Informed consent, patient autonomy, patient rights advocacy, and universal access to healthcare are all part of this.

Phlebotomy technicians have a duty to protect the health of their patients and themselves from the spread of infection. They need to employ good hand hygiene, PPE, and follow recognized methods for controlling infections. Patients and healthcare staff are better protected when standard precautions and infection control procedures are followed.

Key Takeaways of Core Knowledge

Technicians in phlebotomy are vital to the medical field since they are responsible for drawing blood samples for analysis. They should have the knowledge, experience, and expertise to collect specimens accurately and safely.

When taking blood samples, it is crucial to practice aseptic procedure to avoid contaminating the samples and exposing the patient to unnecessary infection risk. Proper hygienic practices, including the use of antiseptics and the maintenance of a sterile environment, must be adhered to at all times during blood collection.

Red blood cells, white blood cells, platelets, and plasma are only some of the many blood components that must be understood for correct interpretation of laboratory test results and medical diagnosis.

Transfusion compatibility and the avoidance of adverse responses require an understanding of blood type systems like ABO and Rh. Correct identification of blood types during blood collection by phlebotomists is essential for the safety of transfusion procedures.

Knowledge of vascular architecture aids phlebotomy technicians in finding appropriate veins for blood collection, hence reducing patient discomfort and the likelihood of complications.

Phlebotomy technicians must have a firm grasp of the cardiovascular system in order to fully appreciate the effects of blood collection on the circulatory system and see early warning indications of trouble.

Understanding the mechanisms of hemostasis and coagulation is essential for collecting and interpreting findings from coagulation tests.

Laboratory test findings can be affected by pre-analytical errors, such as those caused by incorrect labelling, hemolysis, or contamination, thus phlebotomy technicians need to be aware of these potential problems.

The Needlestick Safety and Prevention Act ensures the safety of healthcare workers by requiring healthcare facilities to take precautions against needlestick injuries and exposures to bloodborne pathogens.

Care Continuity, Legal Compliance, Quality Improvement, and Research All Depend on Accurate and Detailed Documentation and Reporting.

Establishing rapport, ensuring patients understand and cooperate, and providing excellent treatment all depend on your ability to communicate effectively both verbally and nonverbally.

Chapter 13

Laboratory Information Systems

Today's healthcare facilities can't do without Laboratory Information Systems (LIS), which provide full assistance for managing laboratory data, optimizing workflow efficiency, and elevating patient care. This chapter explores the many facets of LIS, including relevant laws and regulations, regulatory bodies and terminology, quality assurance and control, interpersonal communication and ethics, infection and exposure prevention, emergency situations, medical coding and billing. Professionals in the laboratory can benefit from a more in-depth understanding of the implementation and use of laboratory information systems by delving into the aforementioned areas.

Legislation is essential in the dynamic field of healthcare and technology to protect the confidentiality, integrity, and veracity of laboratory data. The Health Insurance Portability and Accountability Act (HIPAA) is among the laws that have had the greatest influence on LIS. The Health Insurance Portability and Accountability Act (HIPAA) establishes nationwide requirements for safeguarding patients' health information, including laboratory results. It mandates the use of privacy and security measures for the electronic communication of health information between healthcare providers, including laboratories, and their patients.

As another piece of legislation, the Clinical Laboratory Improvement Amendments (CLIA) has had far-reaching effects on how laboratories are run and what they must adhere to in terms of quality. Laboratory testing on human specimens must adhere to CLIA requirements, which are regulated by the Centers for Medicare & Medicaid Services (CMS). Qualifications of staff, quality control, proficiency testing, and patient test administration are just a few of the topics addressed by these guidelines. Laboratories that serve Medicare and Medicaid patients must comply with CLIA requirements in order to be paid for their work.

Moreover, the Laboratory Information Systems for Clinical Trials Act (LISCTRA) is impacted by the Food and Drug Administration Amendments Act (FDAAA). Provisions in the FDAAA ensure the ethical conduct of research and the protection of human participants by requiring adequate recording, reporting, and monitoring of safety during clinical trials.

The laws and regulations pertaining to laboratory information systems are monitored by a number of different regulatory bodies. The Centers for Medicare & Medicaid Services (CMS) is one such organization because it oversees the CLIA program. Laboratory accreditation and quality assurance are CMS's responsibilities. In order to keep their CLIA certification current, laboratories must pass periodic inspections and proficiency tests.

The FDA also plays an important role in the oversight of laboratory information systems. IVD devices, which are crucial to LIS, are regulated by the FDA. In vitro diagnostic (IVD) devices are used in laboratories, and the FDA makes sure they meet safety, efficacy, and accuracy standards.

Expertise in the law is crucial for laboratory personnel who work with computer systems. Protecting sensitive patient information from prying eyes is what the law calls for, and this is where the concept of confidentiality comes in. The privacy of laboratory patients must be protected by stringent rules for maintaining patient confidentiality.

Another crucial legal idea, especially in research contexts, is that of informed consent. In order to obtain a patient's "informed consent," doctors and researchers must explain the procedure's goals, potential side effects, and advantages in detail. Before moving further, patients must willingly express their consent, showing their knowledge and agreement of what will happen.

To guarantee precise and trustworthy laboratory results, quality assurance and control in laboratory information systems are crucial. Regular testing of laboratory equipment, reagents, and protocols to ensure their correctness and dependability is an essential aspect of quality assurance. The performance of laboratory procedures can be monitored and maintained with the help of calibration materials, control samples, and proficiency testing.

Laboratory performance can be evaluated objectively by using a third-party proficiency testing service. Testing the reliability of a laboratory's results requires sending in samples with known values to analyze. Laboratory proficiency may be measured objectively by testing, and weak spots can be pinpointed for further development.

Collaboration, coordination, and the effective delivery of patient care are all facilitated by strong interpersonal communication in the laboratory context. Communication among laboratory staff is essential, as is interaction with clinicians and other healthcare experts. In order to make sound decisions in a timely manner, it is necessary to communicate test results, clarify instructions, and review crucial discoveries. In addition to improving the quality and productivity of laboratory work, effective communication creates a more cooperative atmosphere.

Ethical considerations in laboratory information systems cover a wide range of rules and guidelines for how scientists and technicians should act. Confidentiality of patients, informed permission, data integrity, and professional honor are all important ethical factors to consider. The lab staff has a responsibility to protect the privacy of their patients by restricting data access and sharing to those who have a genuine need to know. Essential components of laboratory ethics include respect for patient autonomy and the ethical conduct of research with human subjects. The integrity of laboratory data, the avoidance of conflicts of interest, and the observance of professional norms of behavior are also critical components of a morally sound laboratory.

Infection and exposure to dangerous materials are also possibilities in a laboratory setting. Therefore, it is crucial to implement stringent infection and exposure control procedures in the laboratory for the safety of the staff, the patients, and the community at large. The risk of contamination or the transmission of infectious agents can be greatly reduced if specimens are handled, stored, and disposed of properly. Protect yourself from harmful substances by always following safety procedures and using protective gear including gloves, lab coats, and goggles. Standard operational procedures, risk assessments, and regular training all contribute to a secure laboratory setting.

Medical emergencies can happen everywhere, including the laboratory and its immediate surroundings, therefore workers there should be ready for them. Accidents, allergic reactions, and other abrupt health crises are all examples of situations that qualify as medical emergencies. Professionals in the laboratory should be well-versed in basic life support (BLS) procedures like cardiopulmonary resuscitation (CPR) and emergency response protocols. Prompt and appropriate medical assistance depends on clear communication with healthcare practitioners and prompt activation of emergency response systems.

Coding in the medical field involves assigning unique numeric identifiers to various medical conditions, treatments, and services. Correct coding in laboratory information systems is essential for getting paid what you're due. Correct coding ensures that healthcare professionals can claim their due compensation from insurance companies and government healthcare programmers for laboratory tests and services rendered. Professionals working in laboratories that do coding must be familiar with coding guidelines such as Current Procedural Terminology (CPT) and International Classification of Diseases (ICD) codes.

Accurate and timely submission of claims for laboratory tests and services rendered is what billing in laboratory information systems is all about. Correct billing practices include collecting data including patient demographics, test codes, and diagnoses. It is crucial for laboratory personnel participating in billing operations to have a firm grasp on insurance regulations, coding standards, and the procedures involved in obtaining payment. Successful billing procedures ensure that the laboratory will be paid promptly and accurately for the services it provides.

Important Legislation

Laboratory information systems (LIS) function within a legal environment that is heavily influenced by significant legislation. Health Insurance Portability and Accountability Act (HIPAA), Clinical Laboratory Improvement Amendments (CLIA), and Food and Drug Administration Amendments Act (FDAAA) are three landmark laws that bear directly on LIS.

National rules for the safety and confidentiality of patient health information are established by the Health Insurance Portability and Accountability Act (HIPAA), a landmark piece of legislation. The HIPAA Privacy Rule specifies parameters for the handling of sensitive patient data. In the context of LIS, this legislation safeguards the privacy and security of patient information throughout transmission and storage. Laboratories must ensure HIPAA compliance to safeguard patient information, keep data secure, and prevent fines.

Medicare and Medicaid Services (CMS) run a federal program called the Clinical Laboratory Improvement Amendments (CLIA). Laboratory testing on human specimens must adhere to CLIA regulations, which establish quality benchmarks. Qualifications of staff, quality assurance, proficiency testing, and the administration of tests to patients are just a few of the topics addressed by these rules. Laboratories must comply with CLIA guidelines if they want their test results to be trusted. In order to receive payment from the Medicare and Medicaid programs, laboratories must be CLIA-certified and undergo regular inspections and proficiency testing.

Provisions pertaining to clinical trials and the regulation of medical products are included in the Food and Drug Administration Amendments Act (FDAAA), a comprehensive piece of legislation. Although LIS may not directly deal with data from clinical trials, those working in laboratories should be familiar with the rules that govern such endeavors. The FDAAA promotes the ethical conduct of research and the protection of human participants by mandating the documentation, reporting, and safety monitoring of clinical studies. Laboratories conducting clinical trials or offering their services to academic institutions must adhere to the regulations set forth in the FDAAA.

Regulatory Agencies

Patient safety and adherence to LIS regulation are two of the most important responsibilities of regulatory bodies. The Centers for Medicare & Medicaid Services (CMS), the Food & Drug Administration (FDA), and the Office for Civil Rights (OCR) are three of the most important regulatory bodies in the United States.

The U.S. federal government's HHS department houses the Centers for Medicare & Medicaid Services (CMS). The CLIA program is one of many healthcare initiatives overseen by CMS. Laboratory accreditation and quality assurance are CMS's responsibilities. In order to keep their

CLIA certification current, laboratories must pass periodic inspections and proficiency tests. Laboratory services for Medicare and Medicaid patients are similarly subject to CMS's oversight of reimbursement.

The FDA is a government agency whose mission is to safeguard the public's health through the regulation of foods, pharmaceuticals, medical devices, and biological products. Laboratory information systems (LIS) are not subject to FDA oversight, however, the agency does play a significant role in monitoring IVD devices used in laboratories. In order to assure the reliability, efficiency, and safety of IVD devices, the FDA has established standards and recommendations in this area. When incorporating IVD devices into a laboratory information system (LIS), facilities must follow FDA regulations.

The HHS Office for Civil Rights (OCR) is responsible for upholding HIPAA's privacy and security provisions. The Office for Civil Rights (OCR) is in charge of investigating allegations of HIPAA violations and ensuring that patients' privacy rights are respected. To safeguard patient information and hold responsible parties accountable, the office conducts audits, applies penalties, and mandates corrective actions. Compliance with HIPAA mandates and the use of proper measures are necessary for laboratories to prevent the misuse of patients' personal health information.

Legal Terms

For laboratory personnel using LIS, familiarity with legal terminology is crucial for navigating the legal landscape and maintaining compliance with applicable laws and regulations. Among the many essential legal concepts related to LIS are privacy, informed consent, and data integrity.

To maintain confidentiality, private data must be shielded from prying eyes. The confidentiality of patient health records is of paramount importance in the context of LIS. To protect patient privacy and guarantee that only authorized personnel have access to sensitive patient data, lab technicians must adhere to stringent regulations. Protecting patient privacy in the LIS is facilitated by using security mechanisms including encryption, user authentication, and secure communication protocols.

The term "informed consent" refers to the practice of gaining a patient's approval for a medical operation or participation in a research project before actually carrying it out. The patient or participant must be given full disclosure of the procedure's or study's goals, risks, benefits, and other options. Research and secondary uses of patient data highlight the importance of obtaining informed consent in the context of LIS. Researchers and clinicians who work with human subjects have a responsibility to preserve patients' rights and conduct themselves ethically by adhering to established informed consent procedures.

The term "data integrity" is used to describe how correct, complete, and trustworthy data is. For

LIS to provide accurate laboratory test results and other patient information, data integrity is essential. Professionals in the laboratory setting are tasked with safeguarding the LIS by implementing methods to deter data manipulation, guarantee accurate documentation, and protect data integrity. Audit trails, access controls, data backup systems, and validation procedures are all examples of measures that can be taken to guarantee the integrity of the data held.

Laboratory practitioners using LIS must be familiar with and abide by these crucial legal terminology. Laboratory workers can deliver ethical, secure, and high-quality services while minimizing legal risks by protecting patient privacy, gaining informed consent, and maintaining data integrity. It is imperative that laboratories comply with applicable legislation and regulations regulated by regulatory organizations like CMS, FDA, and OCR in order to operate within the legal framework and deliver the best treatment to patients while protecting their rights and data security.

Quality Assurance and Control

To guarantee precise and trustworthy testing, efficient operations, and patient safety, quality assurance and control are crucial parts of laboratory information systems (LIS). To guarantee that all procedures within a laboratory are up to par, quality assurance involves constant monitoring and analysis of each step of the process. In contrast, quality control is the process of keeping an eye on things like test results, equipment functionality, and reagent integrity to make sure lab work is done correctly and reliably.

The following are some of the methods used in LIS for quality assurance and control:

1. SOPs, or standard operating procedures, detail the processes and protocols that should be followed when conducting tests, maintaining equipment, and handling data in a laboratory setting. These methods help keep the laboratory running smoothly by eliminating wiggle room for error and promoting uniformity.

2. Laboratory test results can be evaluated for accuracy and precision through quality control testing, which entails the routine analysis of internal control samples or known reference materials. Corrective steps can be done to increase the precision and consistency of testing by comparing the actual values with the intended values.

3. Laboratory participation in external quality evaluation programs is at the heart of proficiency testing. These initiatives supply laboratories with mystery samples; they are tasked with conducting testing and reporting findings. In order to evaluate the laboratory's performance and find areas for improvement, the results are compared to those of other participating laboratories.

4. The accuracy and reliability of laboratory tests rely on the precision and upkeep of the tools and equipment used in the lab. Maintenance helps find and fix flaws that could affect

test findings, while calibration makes ensuring the equipment are set up correctly to measure precisely.

5. Reviewing and verifying test results for completeness, correctness, and conformity to set criteria is part of data validation. This helps guarantee that only legitimate and trustworthy findings are shared with doctors and patients.

Interpersonal Communication

Collaboration, teamwork, and the quality of patient care are all positively impacted by good interpersonal communication in the laboratory. Communication among laboratory staff is crucial, as is interaction with physicians and other medical personnel. The following are characteristics of effective LIS interpersonal communication:

1. Communicating in a clear and precise manner is essential for those working in the laboratory, as it helps to prevent confusion and mistakes. If you want to get your point across to people who aren't scientists, you need to use their language and stay away from jargon.

2. Active listening entails paying undivided attention to the speaker, processing what they're saying, and responding appropriately. To guarantee full comprehension and productive teamwork, laboratory personnel should listen attentively to clinicians' and coworkers' directions, questions, and concerns.

3. Communicating in a professional and respectful manner is crucial to fostering an encouraging work environment and sustaining fruitful working relationships. Communication among lab staff should be respectful, polite, and professional in order to encourage cooperation and mutual assistance.

4. Critical results should be communicated to healthcare providers as soon as possible by laboratory staff. For urgent patient care and decision-making, timely communication of vital results is essential.

Ethics

To guarantee the responsible and ethical treatment of patient data, research activities, and professional conduct, ethics play a crucial role in laboratory practice, including LIS. The following are some of the most important ethical issues in LIS:

1. Protecting patient privacy and ensuring the safekeeping of patient data within the LIS necessitates careful adherence to confidentiality guidelines by laboratory staff. Only those who need access to a patient's records should have that access.

2. Obtaining informed consent and adhering to research ethical rules are crucial whenever laboratory activities involve research or the use of patient samples for study. This safeguards patients' rights and welfare by ensuring they are aware of the study's goals and any associated hazards.

3. Professionals working in laboratories should always be honest and forthright when recording their work and reporting test results. It is immoral to falsify or manipulate data, as this undermines the reliability of medical care and scientific inquiry.

4. Maintaining and improving one's professional competency is an important goal for those working in laboratories. This can be accomplished by regular training and education as well as keeping up of developments in the field. Maintaining expertise in LIS techniques and delivering trustworthy test findings are essential for providing first-rate medical treatment to patients.

Infection and Exposure Control

Preventing the transmission of disease and ensuring the safety of patients and healthcare workers are two of the most important goals of infection and exposure control in healthcare and laboratory settings. Reducing the potential for the spread of disease, effective infection control techniques help keep everyone well and safe. Important methods of preventing infection and exposure include:

1. All patients and settings should adhere to standard precautions, which are a minimum set of procedures for preventing the spread of infection. Hand hygiene, using PPE like gloves, masks, and gowns, safely handling and disposing of sharps, and maintaining good respiratory hygiene are all examples. Standard precautions help prevent the spread of disease in healthcare facilities.

2. Safeguards Against the Spread: For patients with confirmed or suspected infectious diseases, additional precautions based on the risk of transmission are taken. Contact, droplet, and airborne precautions are the three broad classes into which these measures fall. When interacting with a patient or their surroundings, it is important to take contact precautions by wearing a mask, gloves, and a gown. Diseases that are transferred through respiratory droplets necessitate the use of droplet precautions, which entail the wearing of masks and other protective gear. Diseases that are spread by airborne particles necessitate the use of airborne precautions, such as the use of respirators and isolation wards.

3. Proper cleaning and disinfection of healthcare facilities is crucial for reducing the likelihood of infection transmission. The standard operating procedure calls for routine cleaning and disinfection of all surfaces and pieces of equipment. Proper disinfectants

must be used, and the required contact times must be adhered to, for disinfection to take place.

4. Vaccines and other forms of immunization are an important tool in the fight against infectious diseases. The best way for healthcare workers to protect themselves and their patients from vaccine-preventable diseases is to ensure that their immunizations are current.

5. In order to stay abreast of changes in infection control policy and practice, healthcare personnel must participate in ongoing education and training. Hand hygiene, PPE use, and the identification and treatment of infectious diseases should all be part of any relevant training. In healthcare facilities, a culture of safety and a commitment to infection prevention can be fostered by consistent education and training programs.

Healthcare facilities can reduce the likelihood of infections and provide a secure setting for patients and staff by implementing extensive infection and exposure control measures. Effective infection control techniques include conventional and transmission-based precautions, thorough cleaning, immunization programs, and ongoing education.

Medical Emergencies

The greatest possible outcome for patients in the face of medical emergency calls for prompt action. Although laboratory personnel in the medical field rarely provide direct patient care, they nevertheless need to be trained to recognize and respond appropriately to medical emergencies. Important things to keep in mind when responding to medical emergencies are:

1. Medical facilities should be prepared for any kind of emergency by having a well-thought-out emergency response plan in place. Procedures for calling in the ER team, notifying EMS, and coordinating the response should all be outlined in the plan.

2. To give emergency care until more sophisticated medical assistance arrives, healthcare personnel must be proficient in basic life support, also known as BLS. CPR, AED use, and the treatment of obstructed airways are all part of the Basic Life Support (BLS) curriculum. Individuals who have received BLS training are better prepared to take decisive action during medical crises.

3. AEDs, first aid kits, oxygen delivery systems, and emergency pharmaceuticals are all examples of items that should be kept in a lab's emergency supply closet. In the event of an emergency, it is imperative that all equipment is in good working order and can be quickly accessed.

4. Coordination and communication are of the utmost importance in times of medical crisis. Workers in a laboratory should be conversant with the organization's emergency

communication systems and procedures. A coordinated reaction and timely medical interventions are guaranteed when the relevant individuals, such as supervisors, emergency responders, and healthcare practitioners, are kept in the loop.

5. **Reporting and Record-Keeping:** It is critical to accurately record medical crises so that trends can be identified, improvements can be made, and regulations are met. Details of the situation, the steps taken, and the outcome of those steps should all be recorded.

Healthcare practitioners in laboratory settings can contribute to a coordinated and successful response by being prepared, trained, and equipped to deal with medical crises. In order to properly manage medical emergencies, one must be well-versed in emergency response plans, possess BLS skills, have access to emergency equipment, communicate effectively, and keep detailed records.

Medical Coding

Coding medical diagnoses, procedures, and services using a standard set of codes for the purpose of documentation, billing, and reimbursement is known as medical coding. Coding that is accurate is essential to effective communication, fair reimbursement, and following rules and regulations. Features essential to medical coding are:

1. International Statistical Classification of Diseases (ICD) and Current Procedural Terminology (CPT) are two examples of standardized coding systems used in the healthcare industry. Diagnosis codes are assigned using the ICD, while procedure codes are assigned using the CPT. Healthcare providers, payers, and researchers may all speak the same language thanks to these coding systems.

2. Codes are selected and assigned after medical coders analyze patient charts, doctor's notes, lab findings, and other pertinent material. In order to assign codes correctly, they must have a solid grasp of coding standards, practices, and documentation prerequisites. A familiarity with code-specific standards, sequencing rules, and modifiers is required.

3. Coding laws and criteria established by regulatory organizations and insurance payers necessitate precise coding in order to ensure compliance and appropriate reimbursement. By accurately documenting and billing for patient services, you can lessen the likelihood of claim rejections and audits. Accurate reimbursement for healthcare facilities is another benefit of coding compliance.

4. Medical coding is an ever-evolving discipline that necessitates ongoing training and education. Medical coders need to constantly learn new things in order to keep up with the ever-evolving coding standards, rules, and trends. This contributes to greater coding precision, regulatory conformity, and career development.

5. It is crucial to conduct regular coding audits in order to evaluate the precision and

conformity of coding procedures. Coding mistakes, gaps in documentation, and other problem areas can all be uncovered through an internal or external audit. It is possible to monitor and enhance coding performance through the use of quality assurance methods, such as assessments of coding accuracy.

Proper reimbursement, data analysis, and communication in healthcare settings all depend on accurate and compliant medical coding. Health care companies can improve their coding quality by adhering to coding guidelines, monitoring coding changes, providing ongoing education, and conducting coding audits.

Billing

Medical billing is the process of submitting claims to insurance companies for payment of medical services. Timely and accurate reimbursement, financial security, and adherence to billing standards all depend on efficient billing procedures. Important things to keep in mind when preparing a bill are:

1. It all begins with the creation of claims in the billing process. This entails collecting relevant data, including patient demographics, insurance information, and coding specifics. Services rendered, appropriate coding, and payment obligations all need to be reflected in a claim.

2. Once claims have been prepared, they must be sent to the relevant payer in order to be reimbursed. Depending on the choices of the payer, the submission process can be conducted either electronically or manually. Payment delays can be avoided and reimbursement guaranteed if claims are submitted on time.

3. Medical billing is only possible with precise coding and thorough documentation. Professionals in the field of medical coding examine patient data and assign diagnostic and procedural codes accordingly. Services must be medically necessary, and paperwork must meet coding rules and documentation criteria.

4. After submitting claims, healthcare facilities must wait for payment processing from payers. Costs associated with reimbursements include but are not limited to rate negotiations, claim processing, and payment posting. Correctly sending payments to patient accounts and reflecting them in financial records is essential.

5. A claim may be denied for a number of reasons, including incorrect coding, lack of medical necessity, or insufficient supporting paperwork. The timely identification and resolution of claim denials should be a top priority for healthcare companies. In some cases, this may necessitate resubmitting claims or filing an appeal with the payer.

6. Regulations and criteria for billing must be followed, and all billing processes must be

compliant with these. Compliance with legislation, such as the Health Insurance Portability and Accountability Act (HIPAA) and billing requirements from payers, aids in protecting patient information, ensuring accurate billing, and upholding professional ethics.

The financial stability of healthcare providers depends on timely and accurate billing procedures. Healthcare organizations can maximize reimbursement and keep their finances in order if they follow a few simple steps: ensure proper claims generation, timely submission, accurate coding and documentation; manage claim denials proactively; comply with regulatory requirements; and provide ongoing education on billing guidelines.

Questions & Answers

Questions

Chapter 2

1. What is the primary role of a phlebotomist?

    a) Administering medications

    b) Collecting blood samples

    c) Conducting laboratory tests

    d) Interpreting medical imaging results

2. Which of the following traits is important for a phlebotomist to possess?

    a) Good communication skills

    b) Advanced surgical techniques

    c) Proficiency in computer programming

    d) Expertise in pharmacology

3. What is one legal consideration for phlebotomists to keep in mind?

    a) Diagnosing patients' conditions

    b) Prescribing medications

    c) Providing counseling services

    d) Ensuring patient confidentiality

4. Which legal concept refers to a failure to perform duties according to the standard of care?

    a) Tort law

    b) Malpractice

    c) Risk management

    d) HIPAA compliance

5. A phlebotomist's failure to properly identify a patient's blood sample can be considered an example of:

   a) Tort law violation

   b) Malpractice

   c) Risk management failure

   d) HIPAA breach

6. Which legislation protects patient confidentiality and privacy in healthcare settings?

   a) Tort law

   b) Malpractice Act

   c) Risk Management Act

   d) Health Insurance Portability and Accountability Act (HIPAA)

7. What is the primary purpose of HIPAA?

   a) Regulate medical malpractice claims

   b) Ensure patient access to medical records

   c) Maintain the privacy and security of patient health information

   d) Establish guidelines for phlebotomy certification

8. Which of the following is an example of an operational regulatory standard for phlebotomists?

   a) Maintaining a clean and organized workspace

   b) Offering financial assistance to patients

   c) Developing treatment plans for patients

   d) Conducting surgical procedures

9. Which characteristic is important for a phlebotomist to possess when interacting with patients?

   a) Empathy

   b) Mathematical proficiency

   c) Radiology expertise

   d) Coding and billing knowledge

10. What is the recommended method for verifying a patient's identity before drawing blood?

   a) Asking the patient for their name and date of birth

   b) Checking the patient's driver's license

   c) Confirming the patient's social security number

d) Using the patient's insurance information

Chapter 3

1. Which of the following regulations governs workplace safety in healthcare settings?

    a) CLIA Waived Tests

    b) HIPAA Regulations

    c) Operational Standards Regulations

    d) Ethical Standards

2. What is the primary purpose of CLIA Waived Tests?

    a) Ensure safe disposal of biohazards and sharps

    b) Implement aseptic and infection control measures

    c) Monitor and control lab equipment quality

    d) Ensure the accuracy and reliability of certain point-of-care tests

3. Which of the following precautions should be taken to prevent the transmission of infectious diseases in healthcare settings?

    a) Standard Precautions

    b) Hand Hygiene

    c) CPR and First Aid

    d) Disposal of Biohazards and Sharps

4. How should biohazardous waste, such as used needles, be disposed of properly?

    a) Placed in regular trash bins

    b) Stored in an unlocked cabinet for later disposal

    c) Disposed of in designated biohazardous waste containers

    d) Donated to medical research institutions

5. What is the purpose of standard precautions?

    a) Preventing exposure to bloodborne pathogens

    b) Ensuring compliance with HIPAA regulations

    c) Promoting hand hygiene practices

    d) Implementing aseptic techniques during blood collection

6. Which of the following is an example of an aseptic technique used during phlebotomy?

    a) Proper hand hygiene before and after procedures

b) Documentation and reporting of incidents

c) Implementing CPR and first aid measures

d) Compliance with HIPAA regulations

7. What does HIPAA stand for?

a) Health Insurance Precautions and Authorization Act

b) Health Information Privacy and Accountability Act

c) Hospital Incident Prevention and Assessment Act

d) Hand Hygiene and Infection Prevention Act

8. How should incidents, such as accidental needlesticks, be documented and reported?

a) Ignored to prevent negative consequences

b) Reported to supervisors or designated personnel immediately

c) Documented for personal reference without reporting

d) Shared only with colleagues to gather different perspectives

9. Which of the following is an important component of lab equipment quality control?

a) Disposal of biohazards and sharps

b) Hand hygiene techniques

c) Regular calibration and maintenance of equipment

d) Compliance with ethical standards

10. What is the purpose of documentation in healthcare settings?

a) Ensure compliance with HIPAA regulations

b) Maintain accurate patient records

c) Promote CPR and first aid training

d) Facilitate safe disposal of biohazardous waste

Chapter 4

1. Which body system is responsible for protecting the body from external threats and regulating body temperature?

a) Integumentary System

b) Muscular System

c) Nervous System

d) Respiratory System

2. Which system provides support, protection, and assists with movement in the human body?

   a) Skeletal System

   b) Endocrine System

   c) Reproductive System

   d) Circulatory System

3. Which system is responsible for voluntary and involuntary muscle movements?

   a) Skeletal System

   b) Muscular System

   c) Nervous System

   d) Urinary System

4. Which system controls and coordinates the body's activities and functions?

   a) Integumentary System

   b) Skeletal System

   c) Nervous System

   d) Gastrointestinal System

5. Which system is responsible for the exchange of oxygen and carbon dioxide in the body?

   a) Respiratory System

   b) Gastrointestinal System

   c) Urinary System

   d) Endocrine System

6. Which system is responsible for the digestion and absorption of nutrients in the body?

   a) Respiratory System

   b) Gastrointestinal System

   c) Endocrine System

   d) Reproductive System

7. Which system is responsible for filtering waste products from the blood and maintaining fluid balance?

   a) Urinary System

   b) Nervous System

c) Circulatory System

d) Muscular System

8. Which system produces and releases hormones to regulate various bodily functions?

    a) Urinary System

    b) Muscular System

    c) Endocrine System

    d) Reproductive System

9. Which system is involved in the production of offspring?

    a) Gastrointestinal System

    b) Reproductive System

    c) Circulatory System

    d) Nervous System

10. Which system is responsible for transporting nutrients, oxygen, and waste products throughout the body?

    a) Circulatory System

    b) Respiratory System

    c) Skeletal System

    d) Urinary System

Chapter 5

1. Before performing a venipuncture, it is important to verify the patient's identity by:

    a) Checking the requisition form

    b) Asking the patient their name and date of birth

    c) Checking the patient's identification bracelet

    d) Asking the nurse for confirmation

2. A requisition form is used in phlebotomy to:

    a) Record the patient's demographic and test information

    b) Obtain the patient's consent for the procedure

    c) Provide instructions for venipuncture equipment usage

    d) Indicate the preferred site for blood collection

3. Obtaining patient consent before a venipuncture procedure is important to:

   a) Ensure accurate patient identification

   b) Obtain permission to perform the venipuncture

   c) Select the appropriate site for blood collection

   d) Document the patient's medical history

4. Venipuncture equipment includes:

   a) Bandages

   b) Cotton balls

   c) Alcohol swabs

   d) Vacutainer tubes and needles

5. When selecting a site for venipuncture, which of the following areas should be avoided if possible?

   a) Antecubital area

   b) Dorsal hand veins

   c) Wrist veins

   d) Cephalic vein in the forearm

6. The correct technique for performing a venipuncture procedure involves:

   a) Inserting the needle at a 45-degree angle

   b) Anchoring the vein above the intended site

   c) Applying pressure to the site after needle removal

   d) Withdrawing the needle quickly after blood flow is established

7. A requisition form for a blood collection procedure should include:

   a) Patient's name and date of birth only

   b) Test(s) requested and collection date only

   c) Patient's demographic information and test(s) requested

   d) Ordering physician's signature and contact information only

8. The recommended patient positioning for a routine venipuncture procedure is:

   a) Supine position with the arm extended straight

   b) Sitting or reclining position with the arm supported

   c) Prone position with the arm bent at the elbow

d) Standing position with the arm elevated

9. Which of the following variables can impact the success of blood collection?

   a) Patient's hydration level

   b) Patient's age and gender

   c) Time of day and temperature in the room

   d) All of the above

10. When collecting non-blood specimens, a critical consideration is:

   a) Using the appropriate collection container

   b) Wearing gloves during the collection

   c) Labeling the specimen correctly

   d) All of the above

Chapter 6

1. The purpose of using evacuated tubes in blood collection is to:

   a) Collect larger blood volumes for testing

   b) Prevent clotting of the blood sample

   c) Facilitate easier needle insertion

   d) Minimize the risk of contamination

2. The order of draw in blood collection refers to:

   a) The sequence in which multiple tubes are filled

   b) The order in which tubes are labeled after collection

   c) The priority given to different patient samples

   d) The specific order of tube colors used for collection

3. When applying a tourniquet during blood collection, it should be:

   a) Applied tightly to completely occlude blood flow

   b) Left in place for a minimum of 10 minutes

   c) Positioned proximal to the intended venipuncture site

   d) Applied directly over the patient's clothing

4. Palpation techniques are used during blood collection to:

   a) Locate and anchor the vein for needle insertion

b) Assess the patient's pain threshold

c) Measure the patient's blood pressure

d) Determine the patient's pulse rate

5. Which of the following factors is a contraindication for venipuncture?

a) Recent administration of medication

b) Localized infection at the venipuncture site

c) Patient's history of fainting during blood collection

d) Patient's preference for a specific needle gauge

6. An antiseptic agent is used during blood collection to:

a) Sterilize the needle before insertion

b) Prevent contamination of the collection site

c) Numb the area around the venipuncture site

d) Promote vein dilation and blood flow

7. Anchoring the vein during venipuncture refers to:

a) Holding the needle in place during blood collection

b) Applying pressure to the site after needle removal

c) Stabilizing the vein to prevent movement

d) Inserting the needle at a specific angle

8. Problematic patients during blood collection may exhibit signs and symptoms such as:

a) Dizziness and lightheadedness

b) Allergic reactions to antiseptic agents

c) Increased blood pressure readings

d) Excessive bleeding from the venipuncture site

9. Possible complications of blood draw include:

a) Hematoma formation at the venipuncture site

b) Infection transmission from the phlebotomist

c) Fainting or syncope during the procedure

d) All of the above

10. Capillary collection differs from venous blood collection in that it:

a) Requires a larger-gauge needle for sample collection

b) Involves collecting blood from a finger or heel stick

c) Does not require the use of tourniquets

d) Is typically performed in an upright position

Chapter 7

1. Peripheral blood smears are performed to:

    a) Assess the cellular composition of blood

    b) Determine blood alcohol levels

    c) Collect a sample for culture testing

    d) Obtain a specimen for genetic analysis

2. Blood culture collections are primarily done to:

    a) Detect the presence of alcohol in the bloodstream

    b) Evaluate the cellular morphology of blood cells

    c) Identify the presence of bacterial or fungal infections

    d) Measure the oxygen saturation level in the blood

3. When collecting blood cultures, it is important to:

    a) Use a regular blood collection tube

    b) Sterilize the venipuncture site with alcohol only

    c) Collect multiple samples from the same venipuncture site

    d) Follow strict aseptic techniques to minimize contamination

4. Pediatric volumes for blood collection are typically smaller because:

    a) Children have a higher blood volume than adults

    b) Children have smaller veins and limited blood supply

    c) Pediatric samples require less volume for accurate testing

    d) Pediatric samples have a higher risk of clotting

5. Throat cultures are performed to:

    a) Assess the presence of bacteria in the nasal passages

    b) Collect a sample for alcohol testing

    c) Identify bacterial infections in the throat

    d) Measure oxygen levels in the nasal cavity

6. Nasal swabs are commonly used for:

   a) Blood alcohol collection

   b) Collecting sputum samples for analysis

   c) Assessing nasal passages for allergies

   d) Detecting bacterial or viral infections in the nasal cavity

7. Nasopharyngeal (NP) culture swabs are collected to:

   a) Determine blood alcohol levels

   b) Assess the oxygen saturation in the nasal cavity

   c) Detect the presence of pathogens in the nasopharynx

   d) Evaluate the cellular composition of the nasal mucus

8. Blood alcohol collections are performed to:

   a) Assess the presence of alcohol in the bloodstream

   b) Determine the genetic profile of an individual

   c) Collect a sample for culture testing

   d) Evaluate the cellular morphology of red blood cells

9. Special considerations for blood alcohol collection include:

   a) Collecting the sample in a non-sterile container

   b) Using an antiseptic agent with alcohol content

   c) Collecting the sample in a red-top or gray-top tube

   d) Collecting the sample immediately after a meal

10. Key takeaways of special collections include:

   a) The importance of following standard procedures for special collection methods

   b) The need for specialized equipment and training for specific collection techniques

   c) The significance of accurate labeling and documentation in special collections

   d) All of the above

Chapter 8

1. Dermal puncture is a technique used to collect:

   a) Arterial blood samples

   b) Venous blood samples

   c) Capillary blood samples

d) Urine samples

2. Which of the following supplies is commonly used for dermal puncture?

    a) Vacutainer tubes

    b) Needles with wings

    c) Alcohol swabs

    d) Tourniquets

3. The primary site for dermal puncture is:

    a) Antecubital fossa

    b) Femoral vein

    c) Fingertip

    d) Jugular vein

4. During the dermal puncture procedure, the depth of the puncture should be:

    a) Deep enough to reach a vein

    b) Sufficient to create a shallow incision

    c) Limited to the epidermis

    d) Determined by the patient's preference

5. Special considerations during dermal puncture include:

    a) Avoiding scars and calloused areas

    b) Applying excessive pressure on the puncture site

    c) Collecting blood into an EDTA tube

    d) Releasing the tourniquet before puncturing the skin

6. The most common dermal puncture site for infants is:

    a) Heel

    b) Finger

    c) Forearm

    d) Earlobe

7. Which of the following factors can affect capillary blood collection?

    a) Temperature of the patient's hands

    b) Time of day

    c) Use of an alcohol swab before puncture

d) All of the above

8. When performing dermal puncture, it is important to:

   a) Apply gentle pressure to the puncture site to encourage blood flow

   b) Reuse lancets for multiple patients to save costs

   c) Discard the first drop of blood collected

   d) Choose a site with visible veins for easier collection

9. The purpose of warming the site before dermal puncture is to:

   a) Increase blood flow to the area

   b) Minimize the risk of infection

   c) Dilate the veins for easier puncture

   d) Prevent hemolysis of the blood sample

10. After completing the dermal puncture procedure, the puncture site should be:

   a) Covered with a sterile gauze pad

   b) Exposed to air for rapid drying

   c) Rubbed vigorously to promote clotting

   d) Cleaned with soap and water

Chapter 9

1. Newborn screening tests are performed to:

   a) Monitor growth and development of newborns

   b) Identify genetic disorders in newborns

   c) Assess maternal health during pregnancy

   d) Diagnose infectious diseases in newborns

2. The process of newborn screening typically involves:

   a) Collecting a blood sample from the newborn

   b) Conducting a physical examination of the newborn

   c) Administering vaccinations to the newborn

   d) Performing genetic counseling for the parents

3. Early detection and intervention in newborn screening are important because:

   a) It allows for immediate treatment of identified conditions

    b) It helps parents prepare for future pregnancies

    c) It ensures a higher birth weight for newborns

    d) It reduces the risk of developing postpartum complications

4. Ethical and legal considerations in newborn screening include:

    a) Obtaining informed consent from parents

    b) Disclosing screening results to extended family members

    c) Sharing screening results with insurance companies

    d) Preserving the privacy and confidentiality of screening information

5. Quality assurance and quality control in newborn screening are essential to:

    a) Ensure accurate and reliable test results

    b) Promote cost-effective screening programs

    c) Minimize the number of tests performed on newborns

    d) Expedite the screening process for quicker results

6. International perspectives on newborn screening may vary due to:

    a) Differences in regional healthcare systems

    b) Cultural and religious beliefs

    c) Availability of screening technologies

    d) All of the above

7. Future directions in newborn screening include:

    a) Expansion of the number of conditions screened

    b) Development of non-invasive screening methods

    c) Integration of electronic health records for screening data

    d) All of the above

8. Newborn screening tests primarily focus on detecting:

    a) Genetic disorders

    b) Nutritional deficiencies

    c) Infectious diseases

    d) Developmental delays

9. The recommended time frame for newborn screening is:

    a) Within 24 hours after birth

b) Within the first week of life

c) Within the first month of life

d) Before the age of one year

10. The primary sample used for newborn screening is:

    a) Umbilical cord blood

    b) Saliva

    c) Urine

    d) Blood collected on filter paper

Chapter 10

1. Centrifuging is a process used in specimen processing to:

    a) Mix different specimens together

    b) Separate components of the specimen

    c) Sterilize the specimen

    d) Reduce the volume of the specimen

2. Aliquoting refers to:

    a) Labeling the specimen with patient information

    b) Mixing the specimen with a reagent

    c) Dividing the specimen into smaller portions

    d) Documenting the processing steps for the specimen

3. When handling, storing, transporting, and disposing of specimens, it is important to:

    a) Follow specific temperature requirements for each specimen

    b) Store all specimens in a single container for convenience

    c) Dispose of all specimens in regular trash bins

    d) Keep specimens exposed to direct sunlight for accurate testing

4. Chain of custody is a process used to:

    a) Ensure the accurate labeling of specimens

    b) Maintain the integrity and security of specimens and their data

    c) Determine the appropriate storage temperature for specimens

    d) Reduce the turnaround time for specimen processing

5. Critical values for point-of-care testing refer to:

     a) The values used to determine the validity of test results

     b) The specific range of values indicating an urgent medical condition

     c) The threshold for abnormality in test results

     d) The values used for quality control of testing equipment

6. Distributing results in specimen processing involves:

     a) Communicating test results to healthcare providers

     b) Shipping specimens to reference laboratories

     c) Storing the results in electronic databases

     d) Training phlebotomists on proper specimen handling techniques

7. Key considerations for handling and processing specimens include:

     a) Maintaining proper specimen identification throughout the process

     b) Ensuring specimens are kept at room temperature at all times

     c) Using expired collection tubes for specimen processing

     d) Handling all specimens with bare hands to avoid contamination

8. Specimens requiring refrigeration should be stored at a temperature of:

     a) -20°C

     b) 0°C

     c) 4°C

     d) 37°C

9. The transportation of specimens should adhere to:

     a) Standard safety precautions only

     b) Local traffic laws and regulations

     c) International shipping guidelines for hazardous materials

     d) The specific transport requirements for each type of specimen

10. Proper disposal of biohazardous specimens involves:

     a) Mixing them with regular waste before disposal

     b) Placing them in biohazardous waste containers or bags

     c) Discarding them in recycling bins for environmental safety

     d) Returning them to the patients for disposal

Chapter 11

1. Patient instructions for urine collection are important to:

    a) Ensure accurate identification of the patient

    b) Collect a sufficient volume of urine for testing

    c) Minimize the risk of contamination in the urine sample

    d) Determine the patient's medical history

2. Urine drug tests are performed to:

    a) Assess the patient's hydration level

    b) Detect the presence of specific drugs or their metabolites in urine

    c) Determine the patient's blood type

    d) Measure the patient's glucose levels

3. Patient instructions for stool collection are necessary to:

    a) Ensure the stool sample is properly labeled

    b) Collect a representative sample for testing

    c) Prevent contamination of the stool sample

    d) Determine the patient's respiratory function

4. Patient instructions for semen collection are provided to:

    a) Determine the patient's fertility status

    b) Assess the patient's cholesterol levels

    c) Collect a sample for genetic analysis

    d) Promote patient comfort and ease during the collection process

5. Non-blood specimen collections may include:

    a) Urine, stool, and semen samples

    b) Blood and urine samples only

    c) Saliva and sweat samples only

    d) Hair and nail clippings only

6. Assisting physicians with specimen collection may involve:

    a) Providing emotional support to patients during the procedure

    b) Performing venipuncture procedures under physician supervision

    c) Analyzing the collected specimens in the laboratory

NHA Phlebotomy Study Guide

d) Administering medications to patients during specimen collection

7. Handling and transporting non-blood specimens require:

    a) Storing the specimens at room temperature

    b) Using biohazard bags for all non-blood specimens

    c) Following specific temperature and storage requirements for each specimen type

    d) Transporting the specimens immediately after collection without any storage

8. The primary purpose of patient instructions for urine collection is to:

    a) Ensure patient safety during the collection process

    b) Verify the patient's identity before collecting the specimen

    c) Educate patients about the importance of specimen collection

    d) Promote accurate test results by following proper collection techniques

9. Non-blood specimens are collected to:

    a) Determine the patient's blood type

    b) Assess the patient's liver function

    c) Detect the presence of infectious agents or diseases

    d) Measure the patient's blood glucose levels

10. When handling non-blood specimens, it is important to:

    a) Wear personal protective equipment (PPE) as necessary

    b) Store the specimens at freezing temperatures to preserve their integrity

    c) Discard any unused portion of the specimen after testing

    d) Mix the specimen with a reagent before transportation

Chapter 12

1. The role of phlebotomy technicians primarily involves:

    a) Analyzing blood samples in the laboratory

    b) Assisting physicians with surgical procedures

    c) Collecting blood samples for diagnostic testing

    d) Administering medications to patients

2. Aseptic technique is important in phlebotomy to:

    a) Prevent the spread of infectious diseases

b) Ensure accurate labeling of specimen tubes

c) Maintain the sterility of the collection site

d) Promote patient comfort during blood collection

3. Blood components include:

   a) Red blood cells, white blood cells, and platelets

   b) Oxygen, carbon dioxide, and glucose

   c) Hemoglobin, hematocrit, and clotting factors

   d) Antibodies and antigens

4. Blood group systems are based on:

   a) The presence or absence of specific antigens on red blood cells

   b) The size and shape of white blood cells

   c) The concentration of platelets in the blood

   d) The amount of hemoglobin in red blood cells

5. Vascular anatomy refers to the study of:

   a) The structure and function of blood vessels

   b) The composition of different blood types

   c) The process of blood clotting

   d) The components of the cardiovascular system

6. The cardiovascular system includes:

   a) The heart, blood vessels, and blood

   b) The lungs, trachea, and bronchi

   c) The liver, gallbladder, and pancreas

   d) The kidneys, ureters, and bladder

7. Hemostasis and coagulation refer to:

   a) The process of blood clotting to stop bleeding

   b) The transport of oxygen by red blood cells

   c) The breakdown of glucose for energy production

   d) The filtration of waste products by the kidneys

8. Pre-analytical errors in phlebotomy can include:

   a) Mislabeling of specimen tubes

b) Inaccurate interpretation of test results

c) Improper disposal of used needles

d) Failure to wear personal protective equipment (PPE)

9. The Needlestick Safety and Prevention Act is designed to:

a) Ensure proper disposal of biohazardous waste

b) Regulate the use of aseptic technique during blood collection

c) Protect healthcare workers from needlestick injuries

d) Standardize blood collection procedures across healthcare facilities

10. Documenting and reporting in phlebotomy is important to:

a) Maintain patient confidentiality and privacy

b) Track inventory of phlebotomy supplies

c) Ensure compliance with legal and regulatory requirements

d) All of the above

Chapter 13

1. Which legislation is designed to protect the privacy and security of patient health information?

a) Clinical Laboratory Improvement Amendments (CLIA)

b) Health Insurance Portability and Accountability Act (HIPAA)

c) Food and Drug Administration Amendments Act (FDAAA)

d) Americans with Disabilities Act (ADA)

2. Which regulatory agency is responsible for overseeing the safety and effectiveness of medical devices?

a) Centers for Medicare and Medicaid Services (CMS)

b) Food and Drug Administration (FDA)

c) Occupational Safety and Health Administration (OSHA)

d) Centers for Disease Control and Prevention (CDC)

3. What term refers to the legal obligation of healthcare professionals to provide care that meets accepted standards?

a) Informed consent

b) Negligence

c) Standard of care

d) Liability

4. Which of the following is an example of quality control in the laboratory?

    a) Reviewing test results for accuracy

    b) Performing regular equipment maintenance

    c) Monitoring temperature and humidity levels in the lab

    d) All of the above

5. Effective interpersonal communication in the laboratory setting is important for:

    a) Maintaining positive working relationships

    b) Ensuring accurate and timely test results

    c) Promoting patient safety

    d) All of the above

6. Which ethical principle requires healthcare professionals to do no harm to patients?

    a) Autonomy

    b) Beneficence

    c) Non-maleficence

    d) Justice

7. What is the primary goal of infection and exposure control in the laboratory?

    a) To prevent the spread of infectious diseases

    b) To ensure the safety of laboratory staff

    c) To maintain a clean and sterile work environment

    d) All of the above

8. In a medical emergency, what should be your first priority?

    a) Ensuring your own safety

    b) Contacting emergency medical services

    c) Administering first aid to the patient

    d) Alerting the laboratory supervisor

9. Medical coding is the process of:

    a) Assigning numerical codes to diagnoses and procedures

    b) Verifying insurance coverage for laboratory tests

    c) Determining the appropriate billing amount for services rendered

a) All of the above

10. The billing process in a laboratory involves:

   a) Submitting claims to insurance companies

   b) Ensuring accurate and complete documentation of services provided

   c) Following up on unpaid claims

   d) All of the above

Answers

Chapter 2

1. What is the primary role of a phlebotomist?

   b) Collecting blood samples (Answer)

2. Which of the following traits is important for a phlebotomist to possess?

   a) Good communication skills (Answer)

3. What is one legal consideration for phlebotomists to keep in mind?

   d) Ensuring patient confidentiality (Answer)

4. Which legal concept refers to a failure to perform duties according to the standard of care?

   b) Malpractice (Answer)

5. A phlebotomist's failure to properly identify a patient's blood sample can be considered an example of:

   a) Tort law violation (Answer)

6. Which legislation protects patient confidentiality and privacy in healthcare settings?

   d) Health Insurance Portability and Accountability Act (HIPAA) (Answer)

7. What is the primary purpose of HIPAA?

   c) Maintain the privacy and security of patient health information (Answer)

8. Which of the following is an example of an operational regulatory standard for phlebotomists?

   a) Maintaining a clean and organized workspace (Answer)

9. Which characteristic is important for a phlebotomist to possess when interacting with patients?

    a) Empathy (Answer)

10. What is the recommended method for verifying a patient's identity before drawing blood?

    a) Asking the patient for their name and date of birth. (Answer)

Chapter 3

1. Which of the following regulations governs workplace safety in healthcare settings?

    c) Operational Standards Regulations (Answer)

2. What is the primary purpose of CLIA Waived Tests?

    d) Ensure the accuracy and reliability of certain point-of-care tests (Answer)

3. Which of the following precautions should be taken to prevent the transmission of infectious diseases in healthcare settings?

    a) Standard Precautions (Answer)

4. How should biohazardous waste, such as used needles, be disposed of properly?

    c) Disposed of in designated biohazardous waste containers (Answer)

5. What is the purpose of standard precautions?

    a) Preventing exposure to bloodborne pathogens (Answer)

6. Which of the following is an example of an aseptic technique used during phlebotomy?

    a) Proper hand hygiene before and after procedures (Answer)

7. What does HIPAA stand for?

    b) Health Information Privacy and Accountability Act (Answer)

8. How should incidents, such as accidental needlesticks, be documented and reported?

    b) Reported to supervisors or designated personnel immediately (Answer)

9. Which of the following is an important component of lab equipment quality control?

    c) Regular calibration and maintenance of equipment (Answer)

10. What is the purpose of documentation in healthcare settings?

    b) Maintain accurate patient records (Answer)

Chapter 4

1. Which body system is responsible for protecting the body from external threats and regulating body temperature?

    a) Integumentary System (Answer)

2. Which system provides support, protection, and assists with movement in the human body?

    a) Skeletal System (Answer)

3. Which system is responsible for voluntary and involuntary muscle movements?

    b) Muscular System (Answer)

4. Which system controls and coordinates the body's activities and functions?

    c) Nervous System (Answer)

5. Which system is responsible for the exchange of oxygen and carbon dioxide in the body?

    a) Respiratory System (Answer)

6. Which system is responsible for the digestion and absorption of nutrients in the body?

    b) Gastrointestinal System (Answer)

7. Which system is responsible for filtering waste products from the blood and maintaining fluid balance?

    a) Urinary System (Answer)

8. Which system produces and releases hormones to regulate various bodily functions?

    c) Endocrine System (Answer)

9. Which system is involved in the production of offspring?

    b) Reproductive System (Answer)

10. Which system is responsible for transporting nutrients, oxygen, and waste products throughout the body?

    a) Circulatory System (Answers)

Chapter 5

1. Before performing a venipuncture, it is important to verify the patient's identity by:

    b) Asking the patient their name and date of birth (Answer)

2. A requisition form is used in phlebotomy to:

> a) Record the patient's demographic and test information (Answer)

3. Obtaining patient consent before a venipuncture procedure is important to:

> b) Obtain permission to perform the venipuncture (Answer)

4. Venipuncture equipment includes:

> d) Vacutainer tubes and needles (Answer)

5. When selecting a site for venipuncture, which of the following areas should be avoided if possible?

> b) Dorsal hand veins (Answer)

6. The correct technique for performing a venipuncture procedure involves:

> c) Applying pressure to the site after needle removal (Answer)

7. A requisition form for a blood collection procedure should include:

> c) Patient's demographic information and test(s) requested (Answer)

8. The recommended patient positioning for a routine venipuncture procedure is:

> b) Sitting or reclining position with the arm supported (Answer)

9. Which of the following variables can impact the success of blood collection?

> d) All of the above (Answer)

10. When collecting non-blood specimens, a critical consideration is:

> d) All of the above (Answer)

Chapter 6

1. The purpose of using evacuated tubes in blood collection is to:

> b) Prevent clotting of the blood sample (Answers)

2. The order of draw in blood collection refers to:

> a) The sequence in which multiple tubes are filled (Answers)

3. When applying a tourniquet during blood collection, it should be:

> c) Positioned proximal to the intended venipuncture site (Answers)

NHA Phlebotomy Study Guide

4. Palpation techniques are used during blood collection to:

    a) Locate and anchor the vein for needle insertion (Answers)

5. Which of the following factors is a contraindication for venipuncture?

    b) Localized infection at the venipuncture site (Answers)

6. An antiseptic agent is used during blood collection to:

    b) Prevent contamination of the collection site (Answers)

7. Anchoring the vein during venipuncture refers to:

    c) Stabilizing the vein to prevent movement (Answers)

8. Problematic patients during blood collection may exhibit signs and symptoms such as:

    a) Dizziness and lightheadedness (Answers)

9. Possible complications of blood draw include:

    d) All of the above (Answers)

10. Capillary collection differs from venous blood collection in that it:

    b) Involves collecting blood from a finger or heel stick (Answers)

Chapter 7

1. Peripheral blood smears are performed to:

    a) Assess the cellular composition of blood (Answer)

2. Blood culture collections are primarily done to:

    c) Identify the presence of bacterial or fungal infections (Answer)

3. When collecting blood cultures, it is important to:

    d) Follow strict aseptic techniques to minimize contamination (Answer)

4. Pediatric volumes for blood collection are typically smaller because:

    b) Children have smaller veins and limited blood supply (Answer)

5. Throat cultures are performed to:

    c) Identify bacterial infections in the throat (Answer)

6. Nasal swabs are commonly used for:

   d) Detecting bacterial or viral infections in the nasal cavity (Answer)

7. Nasopharyngeal (NP) culture swabs are collected to:

   c) Detect the presence of pathogens in the nasopharynx (Answer)

8. Blood alcohol collections are performed to:

   a) Assess the presence of alcohol in the bloodstream (Answer)

9. Special considerations for blood alcohol collection include:

   b) Using an antiseptic agent with alcohol content (Answer)

10. Key takeaways of special collections include:

    d) All of the above (Answer)

Chapter 8

1. Dermal puncture is a technique used to collect:

   c) Capillary blood samples (Answer)

2. Which of the following supplies is commonly used for dermal puncture?

   c) Alcohol swabs (Answer)

3. The primary site for dermal puncture is:

   c) Fingertip (Answer)

4. During the dermal puncture procedure, the depth of the puncture should be:

   c) Limited to the epidermis (Answer)

5. Special considerations during dermal puncture include:

   a) Avoiding scars and calloused areas (Answer)

6. The most common dermal puncture site for infants is:

   a) Heel (Answer)

7. Which of the following factors can affect capillary blood collection?

   d) All of the above (Answer)

8. When performing dermal puncture, it is important to:

> c) Discard the first drop of blood collected (Answer)

9. The purpose of warming the site before dermal puncture is to:

> a) Increase blood flow to the area (Answer)

10. After completing the dermal puncture procedure, the puncture site should be:

> a) Covered with a sterile gauze pad (Answer)

Chapter 9

1. Newborn screening tests are performed to:

> b) Identify genetic disorders in newborns

2. The process of newborn screening typically involves:

> a) Collecting a blood sample from the newborn

3. Early detection and intervention in newborn screening are important because:

> a) It allows for immediate treatment of identified conditions

4. Ethical and legal considerations in newborn screening include:

> a) Obtaining informed consent from parents

5. Quality assurance and quality control in newborn screening are essential to:

> a) Ensure accurate and reliable test results

6. International perspectives on newborn screening may vary due to:

> d) All of the above

7. Future directions in newborn screening include:

> d) All of the above

8. Newborn screening tests primarily focus on detecting:

> a) Genetic disorders (Answer)

9. The recommended time frame for newborn screening is:

> b) Within the first week of life (Answer)

10. The primary sample used for newborn screening is:

    d) Blood collected on filter paper (Answer)

Chapter 10

1. Centrifuging is a process used in specimen processing to:

    b) Separate components of the specimen (Answer)

2. Aliquoting refers to:

    c) Dividing the specimen into smaller portions (Answer)

3. When handling, storing, transporting, and disposing of specimens, it is important to:

    a) Follow specific temperature requirements for each specimen (Answer)

4. Chain of custody is a process used to:

    b) Maintain the integrity and security of specimens and their data (Answer)

5. Critical values for point-of-care testing refer to:

    b) The specific range of values indicating an urgent medical condition (Answer)

6. Distributing results in specimen processing involves:

    a) Communicating test results to healthcare providers (Answer)

7. Key considerations for handling and processing specimens include:

    a) Maintaining proper specimen identification throughout the process (Answer)

8. Specimens requiring refrigeration should be stored at a temperature of:

    c) 4°C (Answer)

9. The transportation of specimens should adhere to:

    d) The specific transport requirements for each type of specimen (Answer)

10. Proper disposal of biohazardous specimens involves:

    b) Placing them in biohazardous waste containers or bags (Answer)

Chapter 11

1. Patient instructions for urine collection are important to:

    c) Minimize the risk of contamination in the urine sample (Answer)

2. Urine drug tests are performed to:

    b) Detect the presence of specific drugs or their metabolites in urine (Answer)

3. Patient instructions for stool collection are necessary to:

    b) Collect a representative sample for testing (Answer)

4. Patient instructions for semen collection are provided to:

    d) Promote patient comfort and ease during the collection process (Answer)

5. Non-blood specimen collections may include:

    a) Urine, stool, and semen samples (Answer)

6. Assisting physicians with specimen collection may involve:

    b) Performing venipuncture procedures under physician supervision (Answer)

7. Handling and transporting non-blood specimens require:

    c) Following specific temperature and storage requirements for each specimen type (Answer)

8. The primary purpose of patient instructions for urine collection is to:

    d) Promote accurate test results by following proper collection techniques (Answer)

9. Non-blood specimens are collected to:

    c) Detect the presence of infectious agents or diseases (Answer)

10. When handling non-blood specimens, it is important to:

    a) Wear personal protective equipment (PPE) as necessary (Answer)

Chapter 12

1. The role of phlebotomy technicians primarily involves:

    c) Collecting blood samples for diagnostic testing (Answer)

2. Aseptic technique is important in phlebotomy to:

    a) Prevent the spread of infectious diseases (Answer)

3. Blood components include:

    a) Red blood cells, white blood cells, and platelets (Answer)

4. Blood group systems are based on:

>   a) The presence or absence of specific antigens on red blood cells (Answer)

5. Vascular anatomy refers to the study of:

>   a) The structure and function of blood vessels (Answer)

6. The cardiovascular system includes:

>   a) The heart, blood vessels, and blood (Answer)

7. Hemostasis and coagulation refer to:

>   a) The process of blood clotting to stop bleeding (Answer)

8. Pre-analytical errors in phlebotomy can include:

>   a) Mislabeling of specimen tubes (Answer)

9. The Needlestick Safety and Prevention Act is designed to:

>   c) Protect healthcare workers from needlestick injuries (Answer)

10. Documenting and reporting in phlebotomy is important to:

>   d) All of the above (Answer)

Chapter 13

1. Which legislation is designed to protect the privacy and security of patient health information?

>   b) Health Insurance Portability and Accountability Act (HIPAA) (Answer)

2. Which regulatory agency is responsible for overseeing the safety and effectiveness of medical devices?

>   b) Food and Drug Administration (FDA) (Answer)

3. What term refers to the legal obligation of healthcare professionals to provide care that meets accepted standards?

>   c) Standard of care (Answer)

4. Which of the following is an example of quality control in the laboratory?

>   d) All of the above (Answer)

5. Effective interpersonal communication in the laboratory setting is important for:

>   d) All of the above (Answer)

6. Which ethical principle requires healthcare professionals to do no harm to patients?

    c) Non-maleficence (Answer)

7. What is the primary goal of infection and exposure control in the laboratory?

    d) All of the above (Answer)

8. In a medical emergency, what should be your first priority?

    a) Ensuring your own safety (Answer)

9. Medical coding is the process of:

    a) Assigning numerical codes to diagnoses and procedures (Answer)

10. The billing process in a laboratory involves:

    d) All of the above (Answer)

Secret Key

Secret Key #1 - Plan Big, Study Small And Smart

The mantra "Plan Big, Study Small, and Smart" is the key to unlocking the door to success and accomplishment. It's a way of thinking and approaching learning that can help you establish worthwhile objectives, break them down into more manageable chunks, and maximize the effectiveness of your study methods. Let's examine the parts of this code more closely:

Set yourself some lofty and motivating goals by getting your "big plan" in motion. It's about letting your imagination run wild and visualizing a world that you want. When you think on a grand scale, you unlock your full potential and go beyond your own expectations.

Setting lofty objectives gives you focus and motivation. It sparks inspiration and drives you toward major accomplishments. In order to get where you want to go in life, you need some lofty objectives to point the way.

Make sure your goals are SMART (specific, measurable, achievable, relevant, and time-bound) for maximum success in your long-term planning endeavors. This structure guarantees that your objectives are clear and achievable. Having defined goals and objectives allows you to track your progress and make course corrections as needed.

Learn the Fine Print: Big plans are necessary, but the road to success is often paved with baby steps. When you study on a smaller scale, you break down larger objectives into smaller, more attainable goals. By breaking down the procedure into manageable chunks, you can increase your chances of success and reduce feelings of being overwhelmed.

If you're feeling overwhelmed by a huge challenge, starting with manageable study goals will help you overcome your fears and doubts. The process becomes more manageable and satisfying as you cross off each little step along the way when you break it down into smaller chores. Making even small gains like these can help you gain momentum, and confidence, and ultimately move forward.

Managing your time and resources effectively is essential while studying on a small scale. Determine which issues are the most pressing and consequential, and give them your full attention right now. Focusing on these essentials can help you reach your end objective more efficiently.

If you want to get the most out of your time spent studying, you need to adopt some sensible study habits. Methods that improve understanding, memorization, and application are the focus here.

Smart studying begins with efficient use of time spent studying. Make a study plan that works for you and your schedule. Space out your study sessions so that you have time to concentrate, but take frequent pauses to avoid burning out.

Smart studying also involves engaging in active learning. Participate in the learning process by posing questions, providing brief summaries of significant themes, and relating what you've learned to real-world examples. Participation in the learning process has been shown to increase both comprehension and retention.

To deepen your grasp of the material, you should consult a wide range of sources. Many resources are available, such as books, films, websites, and interactive tools. Learning is strengthened through exposure to a variety of ideas and methods.

The ability to take good notes is essential for efficient studying. Create a method that helps you to focus on what matters most, from the big picture to the smallest details, and everything in between. Make a habit of reviewing and updating your notes on a regular basis to solidify your knowledge and understanding.

Finally, be sure to regularly evaluate your development and solicit comments. By evaluating your progress, you can see where you can put in more effort in your studies. If you want to improve your method, it's a good idea to get some opinions and advice from people in authoritative positions.

Incorporating the ideas of "Plan Big, Study Small and Smart" into your learning process will give you the confidence to set lofty objectives, break them down into more manageable chunks, and make the most of your study time. Taking this course of action will help you stay motivated, keep moving forward, and ultimately reach your goals. Always keep in mind that the key to achievement is a combination of great ideas, baby steps, and diligent study.

Secret Key #2 - How To Make Studying Productive

It's important to make sure you have a good place to study in order to get any work done. Locate a peaceful spot where you won't be disturbed while you work. Make sure there's enough light, a nice chair, and a tidy place to work. A conducive study space will allow you to concentrate on your work with as little distractions as possible.

It is crucial to keep yourself motivated and on track with your studies by setting specific goals. Set goals for each study session in advance and divide major assignments into more manageable chunks. In order to stay motivated and ensure that your efforts are productive, you need to have clearly defined goals.

Make use of active learning strategies to really get into the content. Substitute active participation in the form of summarizing, questioning, and discussing the material for the passive consumption of text or audio. Using this method, you may get more out of your study time since you'll be able to better understand the material, remember it, and put it to use.

Studying efficiently requires careful management of one's time. Create a timetable that takes advantage of your peak concentration times and devote certain blocks of time to studying. Study in shorter spurts and take breaks frequently to avoid burnout. Sort your to-do list by importance and urgency, giving greater attention to the things that really matter.

Using efficient study methods can make a huge difference in how much you learn. Try out different approaches like spaced repetition, active recall, visualization, mnemonics, and practice problems to see what works best for you. Find out how you learn best and make those methods a regular part of your study practice. These methods are useful for learning new material, retaining information, and solving problems.

Focusing while studying requires the ability to block out distractions. Avoid distractions as much as possible by turning off or putting away all electronic gadgets. You could try installing a browser add-on that prevents you from receiving notifications or visiting potentially distracting websites. If you find that listening to music or using headphones helps you focus, do so. Getting rid of interruptions helps you concentrate better and get more done.

Maintaining your emotional and physiological health is crucial to maximizing your study time. Be careful to get enough shut-eye, eat well, and exercise frequently. Taking time off to meditate, practice mindfulness, or do something else relaxing can help relieve stress and restore mental energy. In order to maintain a healthy mentality and avoid burnout, it's important to take breaks from studying and engage in other activities.

Having someone to talk to or work with while you study can do wonders for your productivity. Participate in peer conversations, peer tutoring, and mentorship programs. By working with others, you can expand your horizons, solidify your grasp of key topics, and amp up your enthusiasm for learning. You can improve your own comprehension and spot knowledge gaps by explaining things to other people.

If you put these methods to use, you may make your study time more effective and enjoyable. To maximize study time, it's important to take into account environmental factors like noise and lighting, as well as personal ones like prioritizing self-care and reaching out for help when you need it. With the appropriate mindset, you can unlock your full potential as a student and excel in your studies.

Secret Key #3 - Practice The Right Way

The importance of methodical and efficient practice in fostering deep and lasting learning is emphasized in the book Practice the Right Way. Going through the motions is not enough; proper practice calls for active participation, specific feedback, and deliberate adjustment. Let's delve into this crucial element further.

Before beginning practice, it is helpful to establish specific goals. Identify the precise areas of expertise or knowledge that you wish to hone. Having clearly defined objectives allows you to direct your energy and time towards improving those areas most in need of it.

Next, disassemble the larger task or skill into its constituent parts. By breaking down the ability into its component parts, you may target your practice sessions more precisely. Targeted progress and a deeper comprehension of the whole skill can be achieved by breaking it down into its constituent parts and working on those.

Focus on quality, not number, in your quest for efficient procedure. The best outcomes can't be achieved by mindlessly repeating the same action over and over again. Instead, give your full attention to completing each repeat perfectly. Focus on getting the details right, honing your technique, and making slight gains with each repeat.

Seeking specific critique is a crucial part of improving one's technique. Seek out advice from people who know more than you do, such as mentors, coaches, or industry experts. Their feedback can be used to pinpoint problem areas and gain insight into how to best refine your abilities. If you want to improve, take their advice and use it to shape your training.

The development of skills relies heavily on deliberate practice. It entails carrying out deliberate and organized tasks that force you to perform at a higher level than you currently are able to. When practicing on purpose, it's important to challenge yourself by taking on challenges that are just beyond your present skill level. Deliberate practice allows you to push your limitations, pinpoint your deficiencies, and acquire new abilities.

Establishing a regular schedule for practice is crucial. Create a routine that works with your time constraints and allows for consistent, focused practice. Mastery of a skill requires constant practice. Schedule in unmovable chunks of time to practice and stick to them religiously.

The two most important aspects of any training program are repetition and variety. Muscle memory and brain circuits both benefit from repetition. But to avoid boredom and improve flexibility, you need switch things up during practice. To build a versatile set of abilities, include a variety of situations, difficulties, and/or circumstances.

Finally, keep an optimistic and growth-focused outlook throughout your training. Adopt a growth mindset and view difficulties as stepping stones to success. Keep going even when things get tough, and reward yourself for sticking with it. Keeping a positive and determined frame of mind is important for maintaining one's practice over time.

You can maximize your time spent practicing and speed up your progress if you follow these tips. Goal-setting, skill-division, focusing on quality over quantity, seeking feedback, purposeful practice, establishing a routine, incorporating repetition and variation, and adopting a growth mindset should all be kept in mind. If you train properly, you can maximize your potential for improvement.

Conclusion

Finally, this all-encompassing phlebotomy book covers a wide variety of topics, equipping would-be phlebotomy specialists with the information they need to excel in their chosen career and pass the NHA Phlebotomy Exam. The book breaks down the exam into manageable chunks and covers topics like what to anticipate on test day and how to study effectively.

The first chapter is an introduction to the exam, explaining its format and what students should expect on test day. Helpful advice on how to prepare for the exam and how to deal with test anxiety are included. Exam preparation can be tackled with laser-like precision with the help of the study methods mentioned in this chapter.

The phlebotomist's duties and the qualities necessary for success in the profession are discussed in length in Chapter 2. Tort law, malpractice, risk management, and adhering to Health Insurance Portability and Accountability Act (HIPAA) and operational regulatory standards are all stressed.

In Chapter 3, we address safety protocols and compliance, including OSHA and ANSI requirements for the workplace, the Health Insurance Portability and Accountability Act (HIPAA) rules for healthcare providers, and ethical considerations and quality assurance measures for laboratory equipment. Standard precautions, transmission-based precautions, exposure control, disposal of biohazards and sharps, CLIA waived testing, aseptic and infection control, hand hygiene, CPR, and first aid are only some of the topics covered. In addition, the processes for recording and reporting information are detailed for maximum effectiveness.

In Chapter 4, the reader is given a foundational knowledge of the human body, including its integumentary, skeletal, muscular, nervous, respiratory, gastrointestinal, urinary, endocrine, reproductive, and circulatory systems, as well as their respective terminology and functions. Establishing a firm groundwork for phlebotomy practice, this text examines in depth such topics as blood structure, the coagulation process, blood vessels, and coagulation and hemostasis.

Chapter 5 focuses on patient preparation and includes topics including patient identification, requisition forms, permission, and venipuncture tools. Site selection, venipuncture technique, requisition form requirements, patient positioning, and other factors that may affect collection are all covered. The need of correct and efficient sample collection is emphasized, along with the discussion of special considerations, testing criteria, non-blood specimen collection, and the minimum and maximum collection amounts.

Routine blood collection is discussed in detail in Chapter 6, which includes topics like blood collection devices, device selection, needle gauge sizes and lengths, evacuated tubes, the order of draw, tube inversion, angle of insertion, equipment quality control, tourniquet application and removal, palpation techniques, maintaining skin integrity, assessing venous sufficiency and contraindications, antiseptic agents and application, anchoring the vein, and handling problematic patellas. The methods of capillary collection and bandaging are also discussed to ensure a complete comprehension of standard blood collection processes.

Special collections are discussed in Chapter 7. This includes blood alcohol collection, smears from peripheral blood, blood culture collections, pediatric volumes, throat cultures, nasal swabs, and nasopharyngeal (NP) culture swabs. The information presented here will help readers understand the unique collection processes for which they are responsible.

The methods, equipment, and protocols for dermal puncture collection are outlined in Chapter 8. Dermal puncture-specific factors are also covered, giving readers the information they need to perform the treatment effectively and safely.

The importance of newborn screening and the steps taken to perform the screening are introduced in Chapter 9. The significance of early diagnosis and treatment of numerous illnesses in neonates is emphasized, helping readers appreciate its significance.

The procedures for processing specimens, including centrifugation, aliquoting, handling, storage, transportation, disposal, chain of custody, point-of-care testing critical values, and distribution of results, are discussed in Chapter 10. These essential procedures guarantee precise and trustworthy lab results.

Patient instructions for urine, feces, and semen collection, as well as the handling and transportation of non-blood specimens, are discussed in Chapter 11 as additional obligations of a phlebotomist. As a reflection of the team approach to healthcare, helping doctors gather specimens is stressed.

Terminology, aseptic technique, blood components, blood group systems, vascular anatomy, cardiovascular system, hemostasis and coagulation, pre-analytical errors, the Needlestick Safety and Prevention Act, documenting and reporting, the importance of verbal and nonverbal communication, and professionalism and ethical standards are all covered in Chapter 12 of this book, which is intended for phlebotomy technicians.

In Chapter 13, we dive deeper into laboratory information systems by discussing pertinent legislation, regulatory agencies, legal terminologies, quality assurance and control, interpersonal communication, ethics, infection and exposure control, emergency situations, medical coding, and billing. Understanding the role of phlebotomy and how it fits into the greater healthcare system is greatly aided by this chapter.

Finally, the bonus chapter provides the keys of successful study, such as how to plan ahead, study efficiently, and practice effectively. These tips will help students improve their study routines and study strategies for higher test scores.

All the topics you'll need to know for your phlebotomy certification exam and beyond are included in this comprehensive guide, including professional obligations, safety measures, patient preparation, collection techniques, processing, additional roles, core knowledge, and larger healthcare issues. The information in this book will provide readers with the knowledge and skills they need to succeed on the NHA Phlebotomy Exam and in their phlebotomy careers.

Made in the USA
Las Vegas, NV
11 April 2024

88506843R00118